PEDIATRIC
NURSING

Mosby's
Review Series

PEDIATRIC NURSING

Paulette D. Rollant, PhD, MSN, RN, CCRN
President, Multi-Resources, Inc.
Grantville, Georgia

Joyce J. Hamlin, MSN, RN, CNS, C
Nurse Educator
Helene Fuld School of Nursing
Trenton, New Jersey

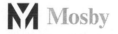 Mosby

St. Louis Baltimore Boston Carlsbad Chicago Naples New York Philadelphia Portland
London Madrid Mexico City Singapore Sydney Tokyo Toronto Wiesbaden

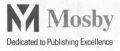

Mosby

Dedicated to Publishing Excellence

A Times Mirror
Company

Vice-President and Publisher: Nancy L. Coon
Senior Editor: Susan R. Epstein
Associate Developmental Editor: Laurie K. Muench
Project Manager: Carol Sullivan Weis
Designer: Sheilah Barrett
Manufacturing Supervisor: Karen Lewis
Cover Illustrator: Susan Swan

Printed in the United States of America
Composition by Shepherd, Inc.
Printing/binding by R.R. Donnelly

Mosby–Year Book, Inc.
11830 Westline Industrial Drive
St. Louis, MO 63146

International Standard Book Number 0-8151-7248-6

95 96 97 98 99 / 9 8 7 6 5 4 3 2 1

Maribeth Moran, RN, BSN, MSN, CPN
Assistant Professor
University of Oklahoma College of Nursing
Oklahoma City, Oklahoma

Angela Trudell, RN, BS, MS, PhD
Child and Family Development Educator
Lawrenceville, Georgia

To Dan, Mom, Dad, Joanne, Joe, Alan, and Amy
Paulette Rollant

To David and my family
Joyce Hamlin

▼ ▼ ▼ ▼ ▼ ▼ ▼ ▼ ▼   ▼ ▼ ▼

HOW CAN *MOSBY'S REVIEW SERIES* BE USED?

Mosby's Review Series is designed to help you obtain the most from your preparation and study time for your nursing exams. These books should be used to review essential concepts, theory, and content prior to nursing courses, challenge, certification, or licensing examinations. The review series can be used to prepare for clinical experiences and as a quick reference when providing care of clients. Mosby's Review Series consists of five books:

Maternity Nursing
Medical-Surgical Nursing
Mental Health Nursing
Pediatric Nursing
Nursing Pharmacology

The series is designed to highlight important information related to the specific content. It is not meant to provide a comprehensive, in-depth coverage of the selected area of nursing. The reference list at the end of each book is a compilation of resources used to develop these books. These references as well as other texts should be consulted when a more comprehensive discussion of a particular topic is desired. Use these books to jog your memory, to reinforce what you know, to guide you to identify what you don't know, and to lead you to appropriate sources for more details. If you are in a formal education setting, these books are not intended to be considered as a substitute for attending classes or completing required reading assignments.

Used correctly these books can help you:
1. Increase your ability to prioritize in clinical situations while using the nursing process.
2. Increase your ability to remember essential content.
3. Increase your productivity in studying to leave some time for you and your family.
4. Apply new behaviors for improvement of your testing skills.
5. Evaluate your strengths and weakness related to content areas or testing situations.

WHAT IS UNIQUE ABOUT *MOSBY'S REVIEW SERIES?*

1. Computer disks of exams
2. Comprehensive rationales
3. Test-taking tips
4. Chapter format
5. References for further reading

Computer Disk

Each book in the series has a comprehensive exam on computer disk. For your convenience, the exam is also included in the book. The answers for the comprehensive exams, like the end of the chapter questions, include the answers, comprehensive rationales, and test-taking tips.

Comprehensive Rationales

These include answers and rationales for each option in each test question.

Test-Taking Tips

These tips aid in your decision-making and facilitate the development of your logical thinking for the selection of the correct answers, especially if you have narrowed your choice to two options.

Chapter Format

Each chapter contains an easy-to-follow format divided into five sections:

Study Outcomes: provides an advanced organizer approach to what is in each chapter

Key Terms: includes the most common difficult terms to recall

Content Review: is organized and structured by the nursing process to help you identify what is most important

▼ All information within each heading is prioritized
▼ Nursing diagnoses are prioritized
▼ Goals are client-centered
▼ Client teaching content is focused for in-hospital and at-home clinical settings
▼ Home care content is included
▼ Older adult alerts are included where applicable
▼ Evaluation criteria includes decision-making tools concerning which actions to take when client's clinical status shows improvement or deterioration
▼ Many tables, charts, and figures contrast, cluster, and simplify information for ease of remembering

Review Questions: stand-alone, 4-option multiple choice

Answers, Rationales, and Test-Taking Tips:

▼ Comprehensive rationales: given for each option to explain why it is correct or incorrect

▼ Test-taking tips: give strategies to use in situations such as when options are narrowed to two or when you have no idea of a correct answer

References
Current references are suggested for further study if more in-depth discussion is needed.

WHAT'S IN *MOSBY'S REVIEW SERIES: PEDIATRIC NURSING?*

Mosby's Review Series: Pediatric Nursing covers the pathological entities of children. The chapters are sequenced in a head-to-toe systems approach. The major systems of neurology, cardiovascular, hematology, immunology, and respiratory include a nursing format with the nursing process as the framework. The remaining chapters target elimination, mobility, endocrine disorders, and special needs of children.

ACKNOWLEDGMENTS

I express my heartfelt gratitude to those who have endured with me throughout this publication opportunity for a nursing review series: an adventure from idea to reality.

I especially want to thank the following people:

Beverly Copland, who thought that I had the potential to complete this project and who eagerly gave me tons of strong support in the initial and ongoing book development phases.

Laurie Muench, who picked up the ball in the middle of manuscript preparation and persisted with me through the process to completion of book publication. The response "OK . . . when *can* I expect it?" provided silent encouragement and sometimes comic relief when my mental and physical energies ran quite low. Laurie's thoughtfulness and guidance to help me set priorities were invaluable! I am very grateful and fortunate to work with Laurie.

Suzi Epstein, who was full of enthusiasm and total support from the birth of the idea for a nursing review series to the final publication of the books. Suzi's creativity and suggestions provided essential building blocks in the overall development of the series.

My *coauthors,* for their enormous efforts to produce manuscript content in a short period of time. Their nursing expertise was helpful for the development of the unique aspects of each book.

My wonderful husband, *Dan,* for his patience, humor, support, and love. His faith in my abilities has sustained my energies and maintained my sense of self.

My parents, *Joseph* and *Mildred Demaske,* for their love, encouragement, and prayers.

Paulette D. Rollant

I wish to acknowledge *Laurie Muench,* and *Suzi Epstein* for their efforts and support in the completion of this book.

Joyce Hamlin

CONTENTS

HOW CAN I USE THIS BOOK?

This book is designed to work for you—at your convenience. Read the following guidelines first to help save you time and energy during test preparation. The chapters are designed for short, quick intervals of review. Carry this book with you to catch the times when you are stuck and have nothing to do.

The directions will help you to:

▼ **Maximize your individual performance in review and testing situations.**

▼ **Identify your personal priorities in preparation for testing.**

▼ **Sharpen your thinking and discrimination skills for testing.**

DIRECTIONS ON HOW TO REVIEW

I. Identify your routine for reviewing: the best days, the best time of day

   A. Write the days and times on the inside front cover of this book and on your personal calendar and the calendar at home. This communicates to your family or support systems that you will be unavailable to them at these times. It is also a nice reminder every week to yourself that this is important to you.

   B. Refer to section V for specific directions on how to develop your routine

II. Scan the table of contents

   A. Put a check mark in front of the content with which you are comfortable

   B. Circle the content in which you think you are weak

   C. Prioritize the weak content with #1 being the weakest content area. Put these numbers in front of your circles.

   D. Prioritize the strongest content areas in the same manner

III. When you are feeling a high-energy day

   A. Go to the #1 chapter of the weakest content area for review

IV. When you are having a low-energy day

   A. Go to the #1 chapter of the strongest content area for review

V. General guidelines for the development of a routine for reviewing
   A. Develop a system of review that meets your needs
   B. Set aside time when you are least tired or stressed both mentally and physically
   C. Limit your review time to a maximum of 90 minutes for the most effective, efficient retention of reviewed content
   D. If possible, relax and take a nap after reviewing to further place the information into long term memory. Some research reveals that sleeping for 2 to 3 hours after studying results in a 70 to 80% retention rate of content into long term memory in contrast to 30 to 40% retention when you are active after studying.
   E. Use at least one relaxation technique *at the onset* and *at the end* of your review time. Deep breathing that is slow with a concentration on the air movement going in and out is one of the best ways to relax physically and mentally.
   F. Use at least one relaxation technique *during* the time you review.
   G. If your time is limited, use 10 to 15 minute intervals to review small portions of the content. For example, you may want to review the different aspects of hypertension in one study session.
   H. Use a theme per week or per day approach. For example, if there is enough time between your test and when you begin to study, every Monday review something on sodium from the book. Then at work find clients with sodium imbalances, review their charts, and discuss their situations with colleagues or with the clients' physicians. Continue with themes for the day such as:
      1. Tuesdays are potassium
      2. Wednesdays are calcium
      3. Thursdays are magnesium
      4. Fridays are acidosis situations
      5. Saturdays are alkalosis days
      6. Sundays are fun days. Don't forget to keep one day to relax and have fun. This allows your mind to work for retention and reorganization of the content that you reviewed during the week.
      7. Weekly themes also might be of help. Do one system per week such as pulmonary, endocrine and so forth.

DIRECTIONS ON HOW TO USE THIS BOOK FOR SUCCESS

I. Suggested study sequence #1 for each chapter
   A. Read the objectives
   B. Complete the key terms

    C. Complete the content review
    D. Complete the review questions
    E. Review the answers, rationales, test-taking tips

II. Suggested study sequence #2 for each chapter
    A. Complete the review questions
    B. Review the answers, rationales, test-taking tips
    C. Review the missed content areas
    D. Review the unfamiliar and the familiar content areas
    E. Complete the key terms
    F. Complete the objectives to evaluate your level of understanding

III. Suggested study sequence #3 *after* doing #1 or #2 suggested sequence
    A. Complete the comprehensive exam in the book
    B. Correct comprehensive exam answers with review of the rationales and test-taking tips
    C. List content areas missed, then cluster them in terms of similar content
    D. Prioritize these clusters with #1 being the least familiar content
    E. Review additional content as directed by the questions you missed

IV. Suggested study sequence #4 *before* doing #1 or #2 suggested sequence
    A. Complete the comprehensive exam in the book
    B. Correct comprehensive exam answers with review of the rationales and test-taking tips
    C. List content areas missed, then cluster them in terms of similar content
    D. Prioritize these clusters with #1 being the least familiar content
    E. Implement either sequence #1 or #2
    F. Complete the computer comprehensive exam. Note that even though the questions are the same as in the book, you should evaluate how your reading of the questions and options differed as related to perception and consistent ability to identify key words, terms, age, and developmental needs.
    G. Review content as needed and directed from your missed questions on your exam

V. Suggested techniques for use of the objectives during your review
    A. Read the objectives to have them guide you where to start
    B. Put a check next to the ones in which you feel the weakest
    C. Prioritize them with #1 being the weakest
    D. Review the weakest content first or on high-energy days
    E. Review the most familiar content last or on low-energy days

VI. Suggested techniques for the use of the key terms, the content review section, and the exams
    A. Key terms—suggested study techniques
        1. Use a 3 x 5 index card to cover the definitions of the key terms
        2. State your definition out loud

3. Uncover the definition and read the given definition out loud (speaking the content as well as seeing the content will enhance your retention)
4. Write key notes in terms of a few words on a 3 x 5 card for the information you have difficulty recalling
5. Carry the card with you for a few days to review this content again. Suggestion: put the card on your sunvisor in the car and review it at the stoplight or if stopped in traffic.

B. Content review—suggested study techniques
1. Use a 3 x 5 card to cover the content under a major heading
2. State out loud what 3 or 4 important aspects of the content under the major heading might be or ask yourself a few questions about that content heading. Try to state the items in order of priority.
3. Uncover the content under the major heading. Check your information against that given in the book. See what you forgot or added that may or may not be important.
4. Write key notes in terms of a few words on a 3 x 5 card for the information you have difficulty recalling
5. Carry the card with you for a few days to review this content again. Suggestion: carry the card with you to review whenever you get 5 to 10 minutes free.
6. When you practice prioritizing the content you will enhance your critical thinking skills

C. Exam review—suggested study techniques
1. For all tests read all the rationales and test-taking tips for missed and correct questions. These often contain pearls of wisdom on how to remember or get a better understanding of the content.
2. Remember to do a relaxation exercise before you begin your questions and repeat the exercise about every 25 questions
3. When you miss a question ask yourself
   a. Did I not know the content?
   b. Did I misread the question or option(s)?
4. If you miss questions because of a knowledge deficit
   a. Make a list on a 3 x 5 card for 3 to 4 days
   b. Group or cluster the content according to the steps in the nursing process, the content area, or a system
   c. Look up that content
   d. Do not look up content after every practice test. A better approach is to cluster the content and look it all up every

3 to 4 days. With this approach you will have better retention into long term memory and the best recall at a later time.

    e. Try to identify new ways to approach reading questions and their options

5. If you misread the question or the option(s)

    a. Try to identify what key words, timeframes, ages, and developmental stages that you may have overlooked

    b. Try to identify new ways to approach reading the questions and their options

    c. Practice, practice and practice doing questions

    d. Practice, practice, and practice doing relaxation before you begin the practice exam, after every 10 to 20 questions, and then at the end of the exam to refresh your thinking and diminish your tenseness or tiredness.

6. Be sure to do a practice exam with the exact number of questions as your real exam. Note after this exam when you were the most tired, anxious, or nervous. Plan to do a relaxation exercise at these times during the real exam.

7. Your success is directly correlated to your degree of effort to review content as well as relax during the review and exam processes.

SUMMARY

It is hoped that after you have completed your review with the use of this book as your major tool that you have:

▼ Maximized your individual performance in review and testing situations.

▼ Identified your personal priorities in preparation for testing.

▼ Sharpened your thinking and discrimination skills for testing.

Let this book work for you to make it easy, enjoyable, and effective to review at times that are convenient for you. The short, condensed, and prioritized chapter content may spark new ways to develop your skills in critical thinking and content recall.

It is feedback from students, graduates, and practitioners in nursing that prompted the development and publication of this book. We welcome your comments. We wish you a successful career in the nursing profession and hope that *Mosby's Nursing Review Series* has made that success a little easier to obtain!

Essential Elements for Nursing

STUDY OUTCOMES

After completing this chapter, the reader will be able to do the following:

▼ Identify essential elements common to all nursing specialties.
▼ Discuss the priority content for each essential element.
▼ Incorporate the essential elements into nursing practice.

KEY TERMS

Client education	Process of meeting the client's needs for the acquisition of skills, knowledge, or attitudes to deal with a pathological condition in the arenas of primary, secondary, or tertiary health promotion as based on the prior skills, knowledge, and attitudes of the client.
Nursing process	Process used as the basis of nursing practice. It includes five steps: (1) assess, (2) select nursing diagnosis, (3) plan, (4) intervene, and (5) evaluate.

CONTENT REVIEW

ESSENTIAL ELEMENTS IN NURSING

I. **The essential elements**
   A. Nursing process
   B. Client education

II. **Nursing incorporates these common essential elements irrespective of the level, environment, or client population**

III. **The nursing process is the priority common thread throughout nursing practice**

IV. **Client education facilitates clients' behavior changes in areas of primary (preventive), secondary (early diagnosis), and tertiary (restorative, rehabilitative) health promotion**

NURSING PROCESS

I. **The nursing process has five steps**
   A. Assess
   B. Select nursing diagnosis
   C. Plan
   D. Intervene
   E. Evaluate

1. Nurses follow the nursing process sequence in any initial client contact
2. Evaluation of the interventions occurs to determine effectiveness or ineffectiveness
3. If effective results, the client-nurse relationship either terminates or new priorities are set for new client problems
4. If ineffective results, nurses select the appropriate step(s); at this point in the evaluation process, the sequence of steps is a creative process by nurses as dictated by client need
5. If a client has unexpected changes during care, nurses typically do further assessment of the situation before implementing actions
6. Use of these steps is a dynamic, client-centered process
7. Communication is essential in all phases of the nursing process

II. The initial assessment process
A. Includes subjective and objective information
B. Subjective information: elicited by questions such as
1. What is the one item that made you decide to seek help?
2. What is your major problem today?
3. When did this start? How long did it last? What relieved it?
4. Do I need to know any other information that can help me better care for you?

C. Objective information: elicited through the senses
1. Inspection: done initially for the client's respiratory rate, breathing effort, color, and position
2. Inspection and touch: a handshake of the client elicits
   a. Demonstration of respect for the client; reduction of client's anxiety
   b. Level of consciousness and the motor ability/strength of client to initiate an appropriate response
   c. Pulse assessment for rate and regularity if two-handed technique is used
   d. Skin assessment for temperature, color, texture, and moisture
3. Smell for odors: done simultaneously with inspection
4. Hearing: asking the initial questions, then auscultating elicits
   a. Specific information about the client's perception of the problem
   b. Information about the client's emotional reaction to the situation by noting the tone and inflection of the speech
   c. Degree of influence from others based on whether they answer or clarify client's answers to questions

          d. Auscultation typically includes the lungs, heart sounds, bowel sounds, and then any vascular sounds such as the carotid arteries or arterio-venous (A-V) fistulas

     5. Touch: commonly the approaches to other touch techniques such as percussion or palpation are completed by starting with the problem system then moving to the respiratory, cardiac, and neurological systems followed by the other systems

D. In emergency situations, objective information may take precedent over subjective information

     1. Airway, breathing, and circulation, the ABCs, may dictate assessment priorities

     2. Deferment of the history and physical assessment of all body systems may take a secondary focus, with priority actions aiming to support the cardiac and respiratory systems

E. Subjective information is best obtained from the client, the primary source, or from secondary sources such as the caretaker, family, or friends

F. History can be obtained from prior documentation to expedite the initial contact and conserve client energy

G. Results of the client's assessment act as the foundation for selecting priority nursing diagnoses and the development of an appropriate plan of care

H. In acute- and home-care settings, nurses may limit priorities to two nursing diagnoses for a more realistic, attainable, efficient, and effective approach to client care

III. The selection of nursing diagnoses

A. Nursing diagnoses

     1. Are clinical judgments about responses of an individual or family to actual or potential threats to health or life situations

     2. Provide the basis for the selection of nursing interventions or referrals to achieve positive outcomes for evaluation

     3. Are designed with a three-part statement; however, in clinical practice the first part is consistently used, but the other parts may not be required as part of the documentation

         a. The three parts, also referred to as the PES format, are

            (1) P = health problem, stated as a nursing problem

            (2) E = etiological or related factors

            (3) S = the defining characteristics or cluster of signs/symptoms as identified from the assessment data

         b. The words *related to* connect the health problem and the etiological factors

  c. The words *as manifested by* connect the etiological factors and the signs/symptoms

  d. Example: urinary elimination—altered *related to* loss of muscle tone *as manifested by* incontinence, nocturia, dribbling.

  e. A health problem may be an actual or a risk for (formerly potential or high-risk) problem

B. Process to the selection of nursing diagnoses

 1. Assessment data are analyzed and interpreted for priorities in relation to time, for an actual or risk for problem with respect to what interventions are accountable by nursing

  a. In acute care: what needs to be accomplished

   (1) In the next 30 to 60 minutes?

   (2) In the next 8 hours?

   (3) In the next 24 hours?

   (4) By discharge from the facility?

  b. In other settings such as clinic, home, and outpatient care

   (1) What was the priority in the last few visits?

   (2) What necessitated this visit?

   (3) What has changed to require a reorganization of the priorities?

 2. A diagnostic label is selected with or without the phrases *related to* and *as manifested by;* institutional documentation policies guide the specific format for each agency

 3. In most situations, one or two priority nursing diagnoses are appropriate

 4. The ABCs are appropriate to use as a guide for setting priorities

IV. The planning process

A. Blueprint for nursing actions, also called nursing orders or planned nursing interventions, which are

 1. Based on the priorities collected or clustered from the assessment data

 2. Selected in reference to time and resources available

 3. Safe for the client and the nurse

 4. Commonly a combination of independent, interdependent, and dependent actions

B. Involves goal setting for achievement of client outcomes

C. May be done cooperatively if client is able to participate

D. Commonly involves some component of education for a client knowledge deficit

    E. **Commonly dictates client outcomes, which need to be**
        1. Achieved in a set amount of time
        2. Objective
        3. Realistic
        4. Observable or measurable for changes in client's activity, behavior, or physical state
        5. Used as a standard of measure in the evaluation process
        6. Examples
           a. Client outcome: within 48 hours the client will sleep through the night without the need to void
           b. Planned interventions
              (1) Provide use of the bedside commode before bedtime
              (2) Give no liquids after 8:00 P.M.

V. The intervention process
    A. **Actual execution of the planned nursing actions**
    B. **Incorporates supervision, coordination, or evaluation of the delivery of care**
    C. **Includes the recording and exchange of information among different disciplines**

VI. The evaluation process
    A. **Based on client outcomes as identified from the planning process**
    B. **Determination of the degree of effectiveness or ineffectiveness of the interventions taken to achieve the stated outcomes**
    C. **Ongoing throughout the client-nurse relationship**
    D. **Often performed concurrently with other phases of the nursing process rather than as a distinctly individual step**
    E. **May result in the client's reassessment to reorder priorities and set new outcomes, especially if the stated time frame has been exceeded**
    F. **Requires documentation of the date when revisement or resolution of the health problem occurred; may be documented as ongoing**
    G. **Requires timely, accurate, and objective documentation and communication**
    H. **Includes identification of the client's level of knowledge and degree of willingness to change behaviors, skills, knowledge, or attitudes in any of these areas**
        1. Diet
        2. Activity

3. Environment
4. Equipment
5. Medications: knowledge of
   a. Expected side effects
   b. Side effects that are treatable
   c. Side effects to report to the physician and within what time frame
   d. Length for the course of treatment

CLIENT EDUCATION

I. Client education: the process
A. **Integral part of nursing care on either a formal or informal basis**
B. **Incorporates the use of the nursing process**
C. **Requires the use of teaching and learning principles**
D. **Varies with clients according to their life experiences, present situation, and age**
E. **Includes six main steps**
   1. Assessment of client education needs or wants
   2. Identification of priorities
   3. Identification of client goals or outcomes: what is needed
      a. Behavior changes
      b. Skill acquisition
      c. Cognitive or attitude changes
   4. Development of a teaching plan
      a. Development of learner objectives
      b. Determination of the content required for the given situation
      c. Determination of the resources and how to use them
         (1) Identify the available referral support agencies
         (2) Identify the materials available for teaching/learning activities
         (3) Investigate whether there is money available for materials, courses, transportation to and from education classes
         (4) Estimate the amount of time available versus the amount of time needed to implement the teaching plan
         (5) Decide whether the nurse will initiate and complete the education or refer to another support service for the education
      d. Determination of sequence and presentation approach of the content

5. Implementation of the teaching plan over a stated time frame
6. Evaluation of outcomes with revisions or reteaching as needed

II. Client assessments for education

A. **Client's knowledge base. What does the client know? What does he or she want to know? Respect that some clients desire no information and document that response.**

B. **Readiness**
1. Emotional
   a. Which stage of loss does client exhibit?
      (1) Denial
      (2) Anger
      (3) Bargaining
      (4) Depression
      (5) Acceptance
   b. If clients are in denial or anger, education will probably be ineffective; document stage of loss
2. Motivational: intrinsic motivation, stimulated from within the learner, is preferred to extrinsic motivation, stimulated from outside the learner
3. Experiential climate
   a. Values associated with social roles
   b. Personal resources and support systems
      (1) Family, friends
      (2) Finances for medications, equipment
      (3) Environmental factors: indoor plumbing, electricity
      (4) Prior and currect exposure to interactions with the healthcare system and providers
      (5) Availability of healthcare services, time versus distance with available transportation
   c. Developmental stage
4. Physical
   a. Clinical status is stable or improved
   b. Functional abilities
      (1) Hearing, attention span, listening
      (2) Vision
      (3) Touch and manual dexterity
      (4) Reading, level of highest education
      (5) Endurance
      (6) Short-term memory
         (a) Limited in its capacity
         (b) Enhanced if distractions are avoided

         (c) Enhanced if opportunities are given for repeating or rehearsing the information
- (7) Long-term memory
  - (a) Unlimited in its capacity and duration
  - (b) Influenced by the rate at which new information is introduced: the best approach is to introduce one new item every 4 to 5 seconds
  - (c) Enhanced by 20% to 90% if material is incorporated into a story or real-life situation
- 5. Signs of client's readiness
  - a. Beginning behaviors of adaption to the original problem
  - b. Exhibits awareness of the health problem and its implications
  - c. Asks direct questions
  - d. Presents clues that suggest client is seeking information
  - e. Begins to ask questions about how to handle situations at home
  - f. Indicators during a teaching session
    - (1) Client is physically comfortable; basic needs are met
    - (2) Client readily gives attention; eye contact is made
    - (3) Client turns off television or asks visitors to leave

III. Special needs of clients for their education
- A. Interventions for low-literacy clients
  1. Give only simple (basic) information
  2. Present no more than three new points at a given time
  3. Give the most important information first and last
  4. Sequence information in the way the client will use it
  5. Give information the client can use immediately
  6. Use the same words when meanings are the same (e.g., medicine or drug, not both words)
  7. Use small, simple words and short sentences; introduce no more than five new words in one session
  8. Present information at the fifth-grade level or lower
  9. Be concrete and time specific. Example: take two pills at 4:00 P.M.
  10. Ask the client to repeat the information or the skill
  11. Use humor appropriately; be creative
  12. Avoid long explanations
  13. Reward frequently—even for small accomplishments
- B. Interventions for older clients
  1. Priority evaluations
     - a. Establish the degree of functional losses

       b. Identify the degree of social support; lack of social support may be an important determinant in the decreased compliance of older adults

       c. Identify their habit structures

       d. Have an evaluation completed by social services or the business office for the availability of monies

2. Clients with impaired hearing
   a. Use low-pitched voice
   b. Face client when speaking
   c. Use clear, concise terms

3. Clients with impaired vision
   a. Use large print and a magnifying glass
   b. Black on white or black on yellow paper may be easier for the older clients to read
   c. Provide adequate lighting
   d. Have client use prescription glasses

4. Clients with limited endurance
   a. Keep sessions short (10 to 15 minutes)
   b. Schedule the teaching session at a time of day when clients are comfortable and their energy levels are higher
   c. Break down the information into small steps
   d. The initial session should have only survival-level information

5. Clients with memory loss
   a. Provide repeated exposure to same message
   b. Provide cues: visual, verbal, written
   c. Question frequently
   d. Use advanced organizers: "I'm going to tell you 2 ways to give your insulin," "I've told you how to give your insulin by using two methods."

IV. Learning theory

A. Learning theory for adults

1. Adult learner is defined as a self-directed, independent person who becomes ready to learn when the need to know or perform is experienced
2. Adult education is learner centered
3. Adult education is dynamic, interactive, and cooperative
4. The responsibility for success of adult learners is shared by all participants
5. Adult learners
   a. Like to participate in identification of their learning needs, formulation of learning objectives, and evaluation of learning

      b. Expect a climate of mutual respect

      c. Enter the learning situation with a life-centered, task-centered, or problem-centered approach

      d. Are motivated internally to learn in order to increase self-esteem, self-confidence, or seek a better quality of life

      e. See the educator as a facilitator rather than a director of the activity

B. Learning theory for children

    1. Learning programs for children are more subject centered

    2. Design of learning experiences is topic centered

    3. Learning may be more of an external process with emphasis on externally sanctioned approvals for learning such as stars, happy-face stickers

    4. Objective, content development, and evaluation process are teacher controlled

C. Factors that interfere with learning

    1. Nervousness, anxiety, fear

    2. Too much content at one session

    3. Unfamiliar terms

    4. Complexity of the task

    5. Limited time with too much content, results in rushing

    6. Background noise or other distractions

    7. Fear of the task or information

    8. Frequent interruptions

    9. Inability of an educator to listen to the client

  10. Absence of silence

  11. Left-handed student's learning skills with right-handed educator

  12. Client is not healthcare oriented; healthcare educator is

  13. Stage of development; older adults may have the attitude that they have lived more or less successfully with their present habits and there is no reason to change now

V. Tools for teaching

A. Types of teaching

    1. One to one

    2. Group

      a. Homogeneous clients for a topic

      b. Heterogeneous clients for a topic

    3. Programmed instruction

    4. Guided independent study

    5. Lecture

     6. Role playing
     7. Simulation
     8. Case method
     9. Demonstration/return demonstration
    10. Computerized instruction

B. Media for teaching
     1. Printed materials: pamphlets, books, crossword puzzles, study guides
     2. Pictorial materials: coloring books, videotapes, cartoons, flowcharts, slides, posters, overhead transparencies, computer simulations
     3. Visual representations: models, actual equipment
     4. Auditory: lectures, paired and small-group discussion, one-to-one interaction, role playing, cassette tapes, simulations
     5. Tactile, kinesthetic: practice with real or simulated items, manipulating or constructing models, playing games, completing worksheets, drawing, preparing charts, bulletin boards, developing a calendar of activities

C. Factors to consider in the selection of media/support materials
     1. Items readily available within acceptable costs
     2. Suitability: for the purpose of the teaching, to the environment in which the teaching will take place, for the availability of ancillary equipment
     3. Language: appropriate, understandable, and useful to the audience
     4. Materials: accurate and relevant to the intended age group and culture
     5. Print size: readable for the intended age group
     6. Illustrations: accurate and related to the intended audience

D. Nurse as a tool of teaching: the nursing professional should
     1. Show interest, empathy, and enthusiasm
     2. Practice expert listening skills; listen between the lines not only to what clients say, but how they say it
     3. Note clients' verbal and nonverbal communication that occurs; be aware of your own communication style
     4. Take a break when the client indicates a need; vary the schedule
     5. Be creative
     6. Keep language simple
     7. Allow enough time for demonstrations and return demonstrations
     8. Summarize at the end with encouragement for any progress, no matter how small

E. **Evaluation tips for achievement of education outcomes**
   1. Evaluation is an ongoing process throughout the entire teaching session
   2. If periodic reassessment of learning indicates no progress, try a different approach
   3. Ask open-ended questions along with specific questions
   4. Ask clients to evaluate themselves

F. **Intervention tips for different age groups**
   1. Pediatrics: the play approach works best with dolls or models; coloring, comic, or storybooks
   2. Teenagers and persons in their 20s: use peer speakers, entertainment, and peer groups and keep in mind that body image and independence are a priority for these age groups
   3. Persons in their 30s to mid-40s: written materials work well with follow-up time to answer questions or clarify information
   4. Persons from mid-40s to early 60s: a few long, single sessions to discuss how the effects of the health problem will interfere with attainment of or plans for lifelong goals
   5. Persons over mid-60s: use short, frequent, one-to-one meetings with material in larger print and keep in mind that maintaining functional abilities is a priority

SUMMARY

A working knowledge of the content in Chapter 1, the essential elements for nursing, will enhance the application of the remainder of the content in the review series. Most nursing professionals incorporate the two elements into their practice, which is based on the changing needs of clients who pursue the acquisition of healthcare services and actions to prevent pathological deterioration of the body. The nursing process and client education are intertwined in the areas of primary (preventive), secondary (early diagnosis), and tertiary (restorative, rehabilitative) health promotion.

NANDA-APPROVED NURSING DIAGNOSES

Activity intolerance
Activity intolerance, risk for
Adaptive capacity, decreased: intracranial
Adjustment, impaired
Airway clearance, ineffective
Anxiety
Aspiration, risk for

Body-image disturbance
Body temperature, altered, risk for
Bowel incontinence
Breastfeeding, effective
Breastfeeding, ineffective
Breastfeeding, interrupted
Breathing pattern, ineffective
Cardiac output, decreased
Caregiver role strain
Caregiver role strain, risk for
Communication, impaired verbal
Community coping, ineffective
Community coping, potential for enhanced
Confusion, acute
Confusion, chronic
Constipation
Constipation, colonic
Constipation, perceived
Coping, defensive
Coping, family: potential for growth
Coping, ineffective family: compromised
Coping, ineffective family: disabling
Coping, ineffective individual
Decisional conflict (specify)
Denial, ineffective
Diarrhea
Disuse syndrome, risk for
Diversional activity deficit
Dysreflexia
Energy field disturbance
Environmental interpretation syndrome: impaired
Family processes, altered
Family processes, altered: alcoholism
Fatigue
Fear
Fluid volume deficit
Fluid volume deficit, risk for
Fluid volume excess
Gas exchange, impaired
Grieving, anticipatory
Grieving, dysfunctional
Growth and development, altered

Health maintenance, altered
Health-seeking behaviors (specify)
Home maintenance management, impaired
Hopelessness
Hyperthermia
Hypothermia
Incontinence, functional
Incontinence, reflex
Incontinence, stress
Incontinence, total
Incontinence, urge
Infant behavior, disorganized
Infant behavior, disorganized: risk for
Infant feeding pattern, ineffective
Infection, risk for
Injury, perioperative positioning: risk for
Injury, risk for
Knowledge deficit (specify)
Loneliness, risk for
Management of therapeutic regimen, community: ineffective
Management of therapeutic regimen, families: ineffective
Management of therapeutic regimen, individuals: effective
Management of therapeutic regimen, individuals: ineffective
Memory, impaired
Mobility, impaired physical
Noncompliance (specify)
Nutrition, altered: less than body requirements
Nutrition, altered: more than body requirements
Nutrition, altered: risk for more than body requirements
Oral mucous membrane, altered
Pain
Pain, chronic
Parent/infant/child attachment altered, risk for
Parental role conflict
Parenting, altered
Parenting, altered, risk for
Peripheral neurovascular dysfunction, risk for
Personal identity disturbance
Poisoning, risk for
Posttrauma response
Powerlessness
Protection, altered

Rape-trauma syndrome
Rape-trauma syndrome: compound reaction
Rape-trauma syndrome: silent reaction
Relocation stress syndrome
Role performance, altered
Self-care deficit, bathing/hygiene
Self-care deficit, dressing/grooming
Self-care deficit, feeding
Self-care deficit, toileting
Self-esteem disturbance
Self-esteem, chronic low
Self-esteem, situational low
Self-mutilation, risk for
Sensory/perceptual alterations (specify) (visual, auditory, kinesthetic,
    gustatory, tactile, olfactory)
Sexual dysfunction
Sexuality patterns, altered
Skin integrity, impaired
Skin integrity, impaired, risk for
Sleep pattern disturbance
Social interaction, impaired
Social isolation
Spiritual distress (distress of the human spirit)
Spiritual well-being, potential for enhanced
Suffocation, risk for
Swallowing, impaired
Thermoregulation, ineffective
Thought processes, altered
Tissue integrity, impaired
Tissue perfusion, altered (specify type) (renal, cerebral,
    cardiopulmonary, gastrointestinal, peripheral)
Trauma, risk for
Unilateral neglect
Urinary elimination, altered
Urinary retention
Ventilation, inability to sustain spontaneous
Ventilatory weaning process, dysfunctional
Violence, risk for: self-directed or directed at others

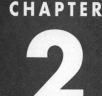

Nursing Care of Children with Neurological Disorders

STUDY OUTCOMES

After completing this chapter, the reader will be able to do the following:

▼ Discuss with colleagues the key terms listed.

▼ Identify the three components of the nervous system.

▼ Describe the various modalities for assessment of cerebral function.

▼ Differentiate between the stages of consciousness.

▼ Outline a plan of care for a child with bacterial meningitis and head injury.

▼ Differentiate among the various types of seizure disorders.

▼ Describe the preoperative and postoperative care of the child with hydrocephalus and spina bifida.

▼ Differentiate between the various forms of spina bifida.

KEY TERMS

Brudzinski's sign	Involuntary flexion of the arm, hip, and knee when the neck is passively flexed, as seen with increased intracranial pressure such as meningitis or cerebral bleeds.
Glasgow coma scale (GSC)	Quick, practical, and standard system for assessing the degree of conscious impairment in critically ill clients and predicting the duration and ultimate outcome of coma. Primarily used in head-injured clients; it involves three determinants: eye opening, verbal responses, and motor responses.
Kernig's sign	Inability to completely extend the leg when the thigh is flexed on the abdomen.
Meninges	Three membranes enclosing the brain and the spinal cord, comprising of the dura mater, the arachnoid and the pia mater (listed external to internal); the arachnoid and pia mater become inflamed in bacterial meningitis.
Opisthotonos	Prolonged severe spasm of the muscles causing the back to arch acutely, the head to bend back on the neck, the heels to bend back on the legs, and the arms and hands to flex rigidly at the joints; more common in children with meningitis or hydrocephalus who are best positioned on their side when this finding occurs.
Reye's syndrome (RS)	Combination of encephalopathy and fatty infiltration of the internal organs that may follow acute viral infections and has an association with the administration of aspirin, especially in persons under 18 years of age.
"Sunset eyes"	Finding in a child with hydrocephalus in which the eyes deviate downward.

CONTENT REVIEW

I. **Overview: neurologic system**
   A. **General concepts**
      1. Structure and function
         a. Neurologic system includes
            (1) Central nervous system, composed of cerebrum, cerebellum, brain stem, and spinal cord (Table 2-1, pp. 50-51)

        (2)   Peripheral nervous system, consisting of motor (efferent) and sensory (afferent) nerves

        (3)   Autonomic nervous system, composed of sympathetic and parasympathetic systems

   b.   Central nervous system (CNS) controls and regulates body functions, including the five senses

   c.   Peripheral nervous system is composed of

        (1)   12 pairs of cranial nerves

        (2)   31 spinal nerves named for the portion of the spinal cord from which they emerge

           (a)   Cervical

           (b)   Thoracic

           (c)   Lumbar

           (d)   Coccygeal

   d.   Autonomic nervous system provides involuntary control of functions, including respiration and digestion

2. Development

   a.   Two thirds of brain cell growth occurs in fetal life; the nervous system continues to grow rapidly during infancy and early childhood and slows during late childhood and adolescence

   b.   The brain and spinal cord are among the first structures to be identified during intrauterine life

   c.   Myelinization—the development of a myelin sheath around a nerve fiber

        (1)   Follows a cephalocaudal and proximodistal sequence

        (2)   Occurs rapidly in infancy and continues throughout childhood

        (3)   Reaches completion in late adolescence

3. Anatomy and physiology: brain

   a.   Bones of the cranium encase the brain; three layers of meninges—the membranous covering of the brain and spinal cord

        (1)   Dura mater (outer)

        (2)   Arachnoid mater—delicate avascular layer

        (3)   Pia mater (inner)—delicate layering that adheres to outer surface of brain. Note: subarachnoid space, filled with cerebral spinal fluid (CSF), lies between pia mater and arachnoid membrane.

   b.   Major structures and functions of the brain are outlined in Table 2-1, pp. 50-51

    c. Brain, blood, and CSF maintain a pressure equilibrium inside skull

    d. Blood supply to the brain is furnished by internal carotid arteries and vertebral arteries, which form the Circle of Willis

    e. Blood-brain barrier, consisting of walls of capillaries in the CNS, functions to slow or prevent passage of various chemical compounds, radioactive ions, and disease-causing organisms from the blood into the CNS

    f. CSF is manufactured in choroid plexus of the ventricular network, which includes

      (1) Lateral, third, and fourth ventricles

      (2) Foramina of Luschka and Magendie

      (3) Aqueduct of Sylvius

4. Anatomy: spinal cord

    a. Vertebral column, consisting of 31 vertebrae, encases the spinal cord; vertebrae divided into segments

      (1) Cervical

      (2) Thoracic

      (3) Lumbar

      (4) Sacral and coccygeal

    b. Meninges cover the spinal cord

    c. Anterior, posterior, and radicular arteries supply blood to the spinal cord

5. Levels of consciousness

    a. Site of consciousness is located in reticular activating system of the brain stem

    b. Assessment of level of consciousness (LOC) gives the earliest indication of improvement or deterioration in neurologic status (Table 2-2, pp. 52-53, and Figure 2-1)

6. Increased intracranial pressure (↑ICP)

    a. Description: condition that occurs when the balance in the volumes of brain, tissues, CSF, and blood is disrupted

    b. Causes: tumors, bleeding, infection, edema of cerebral tissue, accumulation of CSF in ventricular system

    c. Manifestations of increased ICP vary with age (Box 2-1, p. 47)

B. Assessment of the neurologic system

1. Pediatric considerations

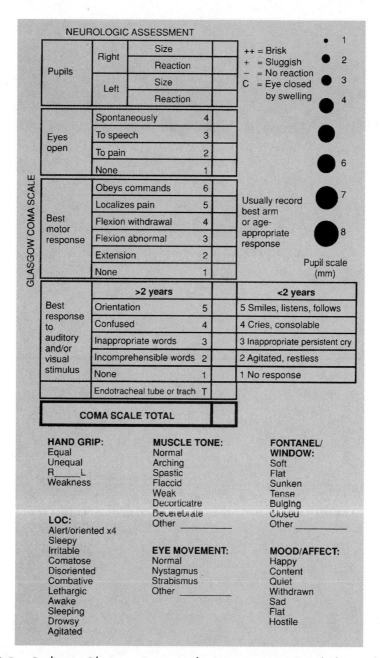

Figure 2-1. Pediatric Glasgow Coma Scale. (From Wong, D: *Whaley and Wong's nursing care of infants and children*, ed 5, St Louis, 1995, Mosby.)

a. Congenital defects of the CNS are mostly the result of failures that occur during the critical period of organ development in the first trimester of intrauterine life

b. Since children less than 2 years of age are unable to follow directions, observations of the level of consciousness and the reflex responses are used to gain information about neurologic status

2. Neurologic diagnostic procedures (Table 2-3, pp. 54-55)

3. Health history

   a. Present health status

      (1) Assessment for the following abnormal findings

         (a) Decreased LOC

         (b) Pain with activity; headache; pain in eyes or ears

         (c) Loss of balance, vertigo, dizziness, unexplained falling

         (d) Weakness or numbness

         (e) School or learning difficulties

         (f) Seizure activity

      (2) Specific questions

         (a) Has parent noticed any clumsiness, drowsiness, confusion, unsteady gait, or muscular weakness?

         (b) Has child experienced learning or school difficulty associated with attention to the task, interest, or ability to concentrate?

         (c) Has the child continued to grow and mature normally?

         (d) Is the child currently taking any medications?

         (e) Are the child's immunizations up to date?

   b. Medical history (areas of concern)

      (1) Prenatal history

         (a) Exposure to teratogens

         (b) Medications taken

         (c) Drug or alcohol use

      (2) Birth history

         (a) Apgar score, fetal distress

         (b) Gestational age

         (c) Congenital anomalies

      (3) Postnatal development

         (a) Infections

         (b) Nutritional status

        (4) Developmental milestones
           (a) Age client attained each of the following: head control, grasping, sitting, crawling, walking, toilet control
           (b) Speech or language: first words, progression to phrases and sentences vs. age at the time
           (c) Performance of self-care activities
        (5) Trauma
           (a) Head, spinal cord injuries
           (b) Birth trauma
           (c) CNS insult
        (6) Infection
           (a) Meningitis
           (b) Encephalitis
        (7) Neurologic or psychiatric disorders
           (a) Hyperactivity
           (b) Autism
           (c) Seizure activity
        (8) Specific questions to ask
           (a) Has the child had a head injury or neurological problems such as seizure, tremor, or weakness in the past?
           (b) Was there a history of prolonged labor or fetal distress?
    c. Family history
        (1) Hereditary disorders
           (a) Muscular dystrophy
           (b) Huntington chorea
           (c) Tay Sach disease
        (2) Neurologic disorders
           (a) Epilepsy
           (b) Seizure disorder
           (c) Mental retardation
4. Physical examination
    a. Mental status
        (1) Physical appearance and behavior
        (2) Level of consciousness
        (3) Attention span
        (4) Memory
        (5) Signs of anxiety or depression
        (6) Speech and language
    b. Cranial nerve testing

      c. Cerebellar function and proprioception
- (1) Evaluate coordination and fine motor skills
  - (a) Spontaneous activity
  - (b) Symmetry
  - (c) Smoothness of movement
- (2) Evaluate balance using Romberg test
- (3) Observe child's gait

      d. Sensory function: evaluation of sensory responses
- (1) Light touch—cotton ball stroked lightly across the cheek
- (2) Pain—skin lightly pricked with safety pin

      e. Muscular function: evaluation of muscle tone
- (1) Pull infant to sitting position using wrists
- (2) Use range of motion techniques

      f. Reflex testing
- (1) Superficial and deep tendon reflexes normally not tested in infants and young children
- (2) Evaluation of common infant reflexes

    5. Relevant medications (Table 2-4, pp. 56-59)
- a. Anticonvulsant: carbamazinepine (Tegretol), phenobarbital (Luminal), phenytoin (Dilantin)
- b. Antibiotics: penicillin G, methicillin
- c. See specific disorder for additional medication information

II. Congenital disorders involving the CNS

A. Hydrocephalus

1. Definition: imbalance of CSF absorption or production, caused by malformations, tumors, hemorrhage, infections, or trauma, resulting in head enlargement and increased ICP
2. Two types of hydrocephalus
   - a. Communicating
     - (1) Occurs as result of impaired absorption within subarachnoid space
     - (2) Referred to as extraventricular—no interference of CSF within the ventricular system
   - b. Noncommunicating
     - (1) Obstruction of flow of CSF within the ventricular system—in the ventricles or from the ventricles to the subarachnoid space
     - (2) Usually the result of a malformation

3. Etiology and incidence
   a. Results from overproduction, obstruction, or malabsorption of CSF
   b. Most common cause of enlarged head circumference in children
   c. Associated with other congenital anomalies such as neural tube defects
4. Pathophysiology
   a. CSF imbalance causes ventricular accumulation of CSF and pressure, resulting in dilation of ventricles and skull enlargement
   b. Complications
      (1) Increased ICP
      (2) Infection
      (3) Developmental delays
      (4) Obstruction of shunt
      (5) Skin breakdown
      (6) Sensory deficits
      (7) Mental retardation in various degrees
      (8) Seizure activity
5. Assessment
   a. Questions to ask
      (1) Any changes in activity level or level of consciousness?
      (2) Any difficulties encountered with feeding?
      (3) Any increases in head size or changes in fontanels noted?
   b. Assessment findings
      (1) Infant
          (a) Irritability and lethargy
          (b) Progressive enlargement of head before fusion of cranial sutures
          (c) Bulging fontanels
          (d) Frontal bossing—prominent forehead
          (e) Distention of superficial scalp veins
          (f) "Sunset eyes"
          (g) High, shrill cry and seizure activity are late signs
      (2) Older child
          (a) Headache
          (b) Nausea and vomiting
          (c) Spasticity of lower extremities
          (d) Altered school performance

     c. Diagnostic evaluation: diagnostic studies
       (1) Transillumination of the skull—in advanced cases, reveals light over the entire cranium
       (2) Skull radiograph—reveals widened fontanels and sutures
       (3) Computerized tomography (CT scan)—reveals fluid accumulation

6. Therapeutic management
   a. Medications
     (1) Diuretics: acetazolamide (Diamox) to decrease CSF production
     (2) Anticonvulsant: to limit seizure activity
     (3) Antibiotics: to treat infection, based on culture and sensitivity results
   b. Treatments: ventricular taps until surgery
   c. Surgery: mechanical shunt insertion into one of the lateral ventricles, usually the right ventricle; distal end placement into another body cavity to drain off excess CSF. Two types of shunts
     (1) Ventriculoperitoneal (V-P)—CSF drains into peritoneal cavity from the lateral ventricle; used most often (Figure 2-2)

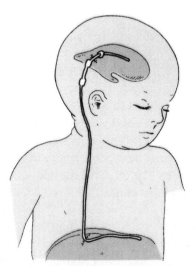

Figure 2-2. V-P shunt. (From Wong, D: *Whaley and Wong's nursing care of infants and children*, ed 5, St Louis, 1995, Mosby.)

        (2)   Atrioventricular (A-V)—CSF drains into right atrium of the heart from the lateral ventricle, bypassing the obstruction

7. Nursing management
   a. Acute care: presurgical
      (1) Nursing diagnosis: risk for injury
      (2) Expected outcomes
         (a) Potential for injury will be reduced
         (b) Skin integrity will remain intact
         (c) Family will be able to discuss hydrocephalus, presurgical procedures, and shunting treatment
      (3) Interventions
         (a) Assess for signs of increased ICP: evaluate LOC using pediatric Glasgow coma scale (see Figure 8-1)
         (b) Monitor vital signs
         (c) Measure head circumference daily
         (d) Position head to prevent skin breakdown; carefully support head when feeding and turning
         (e) Observe seizure precautions
         (f) Prepare family for upcoming surgery
            (i) Explain procedures and treatments
            (ii) Teach signs of shunt malfunctioning
   b. Acute care: postsurgical
      (1) Nursing diagnosis: risk for injury and infection
      (2) Expected outcomes
         (a) Incisional healing without signs of infection
         (b) Potential for additional injuries to head
      (3) Interventions
         (a) Monitor vital signs and neurologic status and assess for increased ICP
         (b) Monitor and report signs of infection
         (c) Place on nonoperative side; position according to physician's orders
            (i) Child kept flat to avoid rapid reduction of intracranial fluid
            (ii) If increased ICP present, surgeon will order head of the bed to be elevated to 15 to 30 degrees to enhance gravity flow through the shunt
         (d) Monitor I&O; maintain NPO as ordered
   c. Home care
      (1) Nursing diagnosis: knowledge deficit

            (2) Expected outcomes
- (a) Family verbalizes the purpose of the shunt
- (b) Family discusses signs of shunt malfunction before discharge
- (c) Family complies with follow-up visits to physician

            (3) Interventions
- (a) Teach family how shunt works
- (b) Teach family signs of increased ICP and shunt malfunctioning and when to notify physician
- (c) Provide information to family regarding support groups such as National Hydrocephalus Foundation, community resources, promotion of growth and development

8. Evaluation
   a. Questions to ask client's family
      (1) What are signs of shunt malfunction?
      (2) What are findings of increased ICP?
      (3) When would you call the physician or take the child to the emergency department?
   b. Evaluation of expected outcomes
      (1) Child remains free of infection and signs of increased ICP
      (2) Parents verbalize understanding of discharge teaching: signs of infection and increased ICP, shunt procedure and malfunctioning, methods to promote growth and development
      (3) Child maintains stable neurologic status
      (4) Incisional site heals
      (5) Family utilizes community agencies for information and support

B. **Spina bifida**
   1. Definition: CNS defect that occurs as a result of neural tube failure to close during embryonic development
   2. Common neural tube defects (Figure 2-3)
      a. Spina bifida occulta: posterior vertebral arches fail to close in lumbosacral area
         (1) Spinal cord remains intact
         (2) Usually not visible
         (3) Meninges are not exposed on skin surface
         (4) Neurologic deficits are not usually present

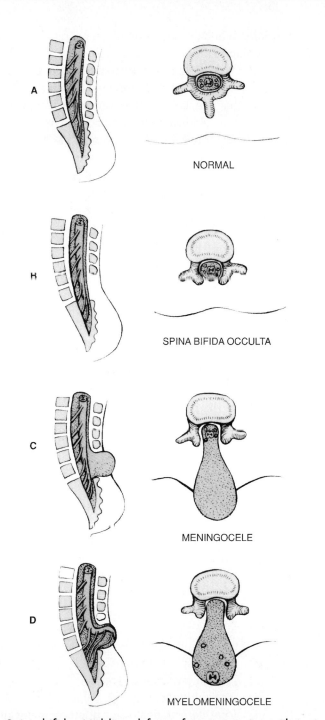

Figure 2-3. Spina bifida. Mid line defects of osseous spine with varing degrees of neral herniations. **A,** normal, **B,** spina bifida occulta, **C,** meningocele **D,** myelomeningocele. (From Wong, D: *Whaley and Wong's nursing care of infants and children,* ed 5, St Louis, 1995, Mosby.)

      b. Spina bifida cystica: protrusion of spinal cord and/or its meninges

         (1) Meningocele—protrusion involves meninges and a saclike cyst that contains CSF in the midline of the back, usually in the lumbosacral area

            (a) No involvement of spinal cord

            (b) Absence of neurologic deficits

         (2) Myelomeningocele—protrusion of meninges, CSF, and a portion of the spinal cord

            (a) Sac is covered by thin membrane that is prone to leakage or rupture

            (b) Neurologic deficits evident

3. Etiology

    a. Specific cause of spina bifida is unknown

    b. Factors involved include heredity, environment, valproic acid (anticonvulsant) ingestion by the mother

4. Pathophysiology

    a. Fusion failure of vertebral laminae of spinal column

    b. Varying degree of neurologic dysfunction present depending on portion of the spinal cord involved: partial to total motor impairment results in flaccidity, partial paralysis of lower extremities, and loss of elimination control

    c. Complications

        (1) Meningitis

        (2) Immobility

        (3) Urinary tract infection

        (4) Mental retardation

        (5) Cerebral palsy

        (6) Epilepsy

    d. Associated defects

        (1) Misshaped lower extremities

        (2) Muscle atrophy

        (3) Hydrocephalus

5. Assessment

    a. Assessment findings depend on spinal cord involvement

        (1) Visible spinal defect

        (2) Flaccid paralysis of legs

        (3) Altered bladder and bowel function

        (4) Joint deformities occur in utero: dislocated hip, scoliosis, kyphosis, talipes valgus or varus

    b. Diagnostic procedures

        (1) Laboratory tests

           (a) In utero: increased alpha-fetoprotein (AFP) in maternal serum and amniotic fluid

           (b) Culture and sensitivity: urine, CSF

        (2) Diagnostic studies

           (a) Transillumination of sac: ability to transilluminate indicates meningocele; inability to transilluminate indicates myelomeningocele

           (b) Computerized tomography (CT) scan and magnetic resonance imaging (MRI): differentiate between various neural tube defects

6. Therapeutic management

    a. Medications

        (1) Antibiotics: used prophylactically to prevent infection

        (2) Anticholinergics: probantheline (ProBanthine)—to improve urinary continence

        (3) Direct-acting cholinergics: bethanecol (Urecholine) to manage urinary incontinence due to contractions of the augmented bladder

        (4) Antispasmodics: flavoxate hydrochloride (Urispas) to control bladder spasms

        (5) Laxatives: biscodyl (Dulcolax) and stool softeners, docusate calcium (Surfak): to achieve bowel continence

    b. Treatments

        (1) Correction of orthopedic deformities: casting, bracing, traction, and surgery

        (2) Bladder and bowel: surgery and training programs

    c. Surgery: defect closure usually done during infancy

7. Nursing management

    a. Acute care: presurgical

        (1) Nursing diagnoses

           (a) Risk for impaired skin integrity

           (b) Risk for infection

           (c) Risk for injury to delicate spinal lesion

           (d) Knowledge deficit

        (2) Expected outcomes

           (a) Sac remains free of trauma and infection

           (b) Family verbalizes knowledge regarding defect and surgical procedure

        (3) Interventions

           (a) Assess spinal column for presence of defect

          (b) Monitor vital signs and neurologic status

          (c) Protect sac: cleanse sac using sterile technique with sterile saline; cover with sterile gauze moistened with solution as ordered (sterile saline, antibiotic, silver nitrate); gentle handling with feedings, diaper changes; avoid pressure on sac; apply protective devices, if necessary; prone or side-lying position

          (d) Observe for early signs of infection and increased ICP

          (e) Prepare family for surgery and related procedures by providing information

    b. Acute care: postsurgical

      (1) Nursing diagnosis

          (a) Knowledge deficit

          (b) Alteration in urinary elimination: neurologic impairment

          (c) Risk for urinary tract infection

          (d) Body image disturbance

      (2) Expected outcomes

          (a) Surgical wound remains intact and infection free

          (b) Parents list methods to monitor child for UTI

          (c) Child exhibits proficiency in self-catheterization

      (3) Interventions

          (a) Assess vital signs and neurologic status

          (b) Monitor hydration: I&O, IV fluids as ordered

          (c) Monitor incisional site for signs of infection

          (d) Monitor for urinary retention and stress incontinence

          (e) Assess child and family's readiness to learn and their knowledge base

          (f) Assess child for signs of a UTI; hematuria

          (g) Perform intermittent catheterization q 3 to 4 hours

          (h) Teach clean intermittent catheterization technique: allow child and family adequate time to practice

          (i) Assist child in establishing an appropriate catheterization schedule

          (j) Teach the child and family to recognize findings of UTI to report to physician

          (k) Administer antispasmodics, anticholinergics as ordered

   c. Home care
- (1) Nursing diagnosis: altered growth and development
- (2) Expected outcomes
  - (a) Parents verbalize knowledge of normal growth and development of the child
  - (b) Parents demonstrate appropriate care for the child with allowances for maximal independence
- (3) Interventions
  - (a) Assess parents' readiness to learn
  - (b) Assess parents' knowledge base
  - (c) Inform parents that overprotective behavior may hinder growth and development
- (4) Nursing diagnosis: altered family processes
- (5) Expected outcomes
  - (a) Family demonstrates ability to safely care for the child with a chronic condition, as well as to maintain usual family functions
  - (b) Family demonstrates effective coping strategies and supportive behaviors
- (6) Interventions
  - (a) Assist family to identify support systems
  - (b) Provide emotional care and refer to community agencies and services, including Spina Bifida Association
  - (c) Provide instruction to family with inclusion of return demonstrations for bladder and bowel training, skin care
  - (d) Encourage maximal functioning with assistive aids for ADLs and mobility
  - (e) Educate parents regarding growth and development
- (7) Additional nursing diagnoses
  - (a) Impaired physical mobility
  - (b) Constipation
  - (c) Body-image disturbance

8. Evaluation
   a. Questions to ask
- (1) What findings should you report to a physician?
- (2) What are problem areas of care or growth and development that you expect or have encountered?
- (3) Do you see any barriers in your home that may hinder the child's mobility?

      b. Behaviors to observe
         (1) Decreased incontinence
         (2) Child adheres to individualized rehabilitation program
         (3) Infection is prevented
      c. Evaluation of expected outcomes
         (1) Presurgical
            (a) Sac integrity is maintained
            (b) Sac remains free of infection
         (2) Postsurgical: surgical wound in the process of healing
         (3) Discharge: family members and/or child
            (a) Comply with daily care and therapy regimen
            (b) Are receptive to assistance from community agencies as indicated
            (c) Integrate regimen for child's care into family routine
            (d) Verbalize normal growth and development behaviors
            (e) Identify rationale for catheterization program and schedule for catheterization

III. Acquired disorders involving the CNS

  A. **Meningitis**
     1. Description—inflammation of meninges, caused by a bacterial or viral infection
     2. Most common bacterial causes: hemophilus influenza (type B), streptococcus pneumonia, and neisseria meningitides
     3. Etiology and incidence
       a. Peak incidence is between 6 and 12 months of age
       b. Primary organism for causing meningitis between 3 months and 5 years of age is hemophilus influenza
     4. Pathophysiology
       a. Organisms invade CNS as a result of trauma or are carried from other sites of infection (such as middle ear, nasopharynx, or sinuses) to the CSF
       b. Aseptic meningitis, caused by a virus, is associated with other diseases such as measles, mumps, or herpes
       c. Complications
         (1) Deafness
         (2) Blindness
         (3) Developmental delay

          (4) Cerebral palsy

          (5) Mental retardation

          (6) Seizures

          (7) Attention deficit–hyperactivity disorder

5. Assessment

    a. Questions to ask

        (1) Have there been recent episodes of middle ear or sinus infection?

        (2) Has there been any recent exposure to communicable or viral disorders?

    b. Assessment findings

        (1) Infants and young children

            (a) Fever

            (b) Irritability; shrill cry

            (c) Lethargy

            (d) Poor feeding

            (e) Vomiting

            (f) Seizures

        (2) Older children

            (a) Irritability

            (b) Headache

            (c) Fever

            (d) Photophobia

            (e) Nuchal rigidity

            (f) Drowsiness

            (g) Seizures

            (h) Brudzinski's sign—the involuntary flexion of the arm, hip, and knee when the neck is passively flexed

            (i) Positive Kernig's sign—the inability to completely extend the leg when the thigh is flexed on the abdomen

            (j) Opisthotonos—severe muscle spasm causing the back to arch and the head to bend back on the neck, the heel to bend back on the legs, and the arms and legs to flex rigidly at the joints; position clients on their sides

    c. Diagnostic procedures

        (1) Laboratory tests

            (a) Lumbar puncture

                (i) Bacterial: cloudy CSF; increased WBC; polymorphonuclear leukocytes, increased protein, decreased glucose, increased pressure reading

      (ii) Viral: slight increased WBC, protein; usually normal glucose and clear CSF

    (b) Cultures: CSF, blood, urine, and nasopharynx—identification of causative organism

    (c) Serum electrolytes: increased Na⁺ and decreased K⁺ indicate dehydration

    (d) CBC: markedly increased WBC in bacterial; mildly elevated in viral

  (2) Diagnostic studies: computerized tomography (CT) scan identifies abscess, effusion, hydrocephalus

6. Therapeutic management
    a. Medications
        (1) Antibiotics: to treat causative organism or prevent opportunistic infection
        (2) Anticonvulsant: to prevent seizures
        (3) Antipyretics: to decrease fever
    b. Treatments
        (1) Correction of fluid deficits
        (2) Electrolyte replacement

7. Nursing management
    a. Acute care
        (1) Nursing diagnosis: risk for injury
        (2) Expected outcome: neurologic status returns to baseline parameters for age
        (3) Interventions
            (a) Assess neurologic status including LOC, vital signs, pupillary response, head circumference
            (b) Assess for seizure activity with implementation of seizure precautions
            (c) Isolate child to protect others from infection
            (d) Provide comfort measures: quiet, calm environment; minimal handling; dim lighting; restricted visitation
            (e) Provide frequent rest periods
            (f) Elevate head to 30 degrees; prevent neck flexion, which may hinder CSF drainage with resultant increased ICP
        (4) Nursing diagnosis: hyperthermia
        (5) Expected outcome: body temperature returns to baseline for age

(6) Interventions
   (a) Assess temperature q 1 to 2 hours using axillary route for infant, tympanic or oral route for toddlers, preschoolers, or older children
   (b) Administer antipyretic as ordered for temperature above 102° F
   (c) Provide tepid sponge baths or hypothermia blanket
   (d) Restrict fluid intake by mouth for first 48 hours to decrease ICP, if applicable
   (e) Maintain IV therapy as ordered
   (f) Encourage fluid intake by mouth as condition permits

(7) Nursing diagnosis: parental anxiety

(8) Expected outcome: parental anxiety decreases with education about the disease process and the course of treatment

(9) Interventions
   (a) Assess family members' levels of anxiety and need for information and support
   (b) Encourage expression of concerns and feelings
   (c) Provide emotional support
   (d) Provide information about the disease process, diagnostic procedures, treatments

b. Home care
   (1) Nursing diagnosis: knowledge deficit
   (2) Expected outcome: knowledge exhibited for safe administration of medications, activity levels allowed, and changes in status for reporting to physician
   (3) Interventions
      (a) Assess educational level of caregiver in the home
      (b) Assess knowledge base regarding disease and therapeutic regimen
      (c) Provide information regarding disease with use of appropriate terminology, pictures, or written materials
      (d) Demonstrate proper technique for administration of medications; explain dosages, times, side effects; provide written information
      (e) Observe parents' return demonstration for correct medication administration technique

(f) Discuss the need for adequate rest periods, rationale for isolation: to prevent spread of disease

(g) Suggest age-appropriate activities to promote stimulation and continued development

8. Evaluation
   a. Questions to ask family
      (1) What precautions will you take to prevent recurrence of infection?
      (2) What findings should you report to your physician?
   b. Evaluation of expected outcomes
      (1) Parent administers antibiotic correctly
      (2) Disease process is resolved without long-term complications
      (3) Family maintains follow-up visits to physician or clinic
      (4) Child demonstrates appropriate growth and developmental milestones for age

B. **Reye's syndrome (RS)**
   1. Description: nonrecurring, noninflammatory encephalopathy associated with fatty infiltration of the internal organs—liver, brain
   2. Etiology and incidence
      a. Commonly follows a viral illness: influenza, varicella (chicken pox), upper respiratory infection
      b. Research has linked aspirin administration and viral infection with RS
      c. School-age period is time of peak occurrence
   3. Pathophysiology
      a. Mitochondrial damage possibly caused by viruses, drugs, environmental toxins, or genetic factors
      b. Encephalopathy is the result of hepatic dysfunction, which causes
         (1) Hypoglycemia
         (2) Increased levels of blood and brain ammonia and lactic acid
      c. Fatty degeneration occurs in
         (1) Kidney
         (2) Heart
         (3) Lung
         (4) Skeletal muscle
         (5) Pancreas
   4. Assessment
      a. Initial questions to ask

        (1) Has there been a recent viral illness such as chicken pox or influenza?

        (2) Has there been any administration of aspirin-containing products?

  b. Assessment findings: divided into five stages of increasing severity (Box 2-2, p. 48)

  c. Diagnostic procedures

    (1) Laboratory tests

        (a) Serum ammonia: increased

        (b) Serum glucose: increased

        (c) Enzymes: increased amylase and lipase

        (d) Serum transaminases: increased SGPT and LDH

        (e) Serum cholesterol: decreased

        (f) PT, APTT: prolonged

    (2) Diagnostic studies: liver biopsy—abnormal results indicate impaired liver function

5. Therapeutic management

  a. Medications

    (1) Muscle paralysis: pancuronium bromide (Pavulon) induces paralysis and relaxes muscles if mechanical ventilation is required; must use sedation such as morphine, midazolam (Versed) along with paralyzing agent

    (2) Anticonvulsant: to prevent or treat seizures

    (3) Diuretics: mannitol (Osmitrol) induces diuresis by increasing osmotic pressure of glomerular filtrate to prevent reabsorption of water

  b. Treatments

    (1) Mechanical ventilation

    (2) ICP monitoring

    (3) Fluid and electrolyte replacement

        (a) Dextrose solution corrects hypoglycemia, which may result in brain damage

        (b) Fresh frozen plasma or vitamin K corrects hemorrhagic complications

6. Nursing management

  a. Acute care

    (1) Nursing diagnosis: altered thought processes

    (2) Expected outcomes

        (a) Restoration of mental functions

        (b) Absence of findings: increased ICP and encephalopathy

 (3) Interventions
  (a) Assess for increased ICP—lethargy, difficulty arousing
  (b) Perform neurologic checks q 2 hours
  (c) Elevate head of bed to 30 degrees, with head and neck in a neutral position
  (d) Provide age- and condition-appropriate stimuli, toys, and activities
 (4) Nursing diagnosis: parental anxiety
 (5) Expected outcome: decreased anxiety as knowledge of disease process and treatments increases
 (6) Interventions
  (a) Assess anxiety level and need for information regarding severity of child's condition
  (b) Encourage expression of feelings with encouragement to ask questions relevant to child's condition
  (c) Facilitate parents' efforts to stay with child
  (d) Ask parents to bring a favorite toy for the child
  (e) Explain rationale for procedures, equipment, and hospital routine
  (f) Update parents concerning child's condition, state of consciousness
 (7) Nursing diagnosis: risk for injury—bleeding, hypoglycemia
 (8) Expected outcome
  (a) Prevention of complications of disorder
  (b) Maintenance of stable neurologic status
 (9) Interventions
  (a) Assess RS stage by noting findings associated with condition
  (b) Monitor blood glucose q 2 to 4 hours
  (c) Administer IV dextrose solution as ordered
  (d) Administer medications, as ordered, to decrease edema, prevent seizures, and decrease agitation
  (e) Seizure precautions
  (f) Monitor for signs of bleeding: increased prothrombin time; stool for occult blood, bleeding or oozing from orifices or mucous membranes
  (g) Administer vitamin K, fresh frozen plasma as indicated

  b. Home care
    (1) Nursing diagnosis: knowledge deficit
    (2) Expected outcomes: family will comply with
        follow-up care and rehabilitation as needed
    (3) Interventions
        (a) Inform parents that deficits generally improve
            and resolve within 6 to 12 months of recovery
        (b) Inform parents of possibility and availability of
            rehabilitation therapy
        (c) Provide referral to local chapter of National
            Reye's Syndrome Foundation for ongoing
            support and information
  7. Evaluation
    a. Questions to ask
      (1) Do you have any additional questions related to the
          disease process, treatments, and prognosis?
      (2) What are your concerns regarding your child's
          current condition?
    b. Evaluation of expected outcomes
      (1) Parents express reduced anxiety regarding child's
          status
      (2) Parents participate in decision making and care as
          appropriate
      (3) Child maintains stable liver, metabolic, and
          neurologic functions
      (4) Parents comply with follow-up care and
          rehabilitation

IV. Seizure disorders
  A. Description: seizures are sudden, transient alterations
     in brain function resulting from excessive levels of
     electrical activity in the brain; may be a symptom of
     another pathological condition, but the cause may not
     be identified
  B. Classified as either partial or generalized, depending on the
     area of brain involvement (Table 2-5, p. 60)
  C. Etiology
    1. Most seizures are idiopathic in origin
    2. Seizures can be congenital or acquired
       (see Table 2-5, p. 60)
    3. High incidence in the first year of life

D. **Pathophysiology**
   1. Level of nerve cell excitability exceeds seizure threshold
   2. Status epilepticus—child does not regain consciousness between tonic-clonic seizures; potential for the following complications
       a. Acid-base imbalances—severe metabolic and respiratory acidoses
       b. Respiratory depression
       c. Tissue hypoxia
       d. Hypotension

E. **Assessment**
   1. Questions to ask
       a. Have any unusual behaviors been noted: irritability, poor feeding, tugging at ear? How long ago? Is there a pattern of occurrence?
       b. Is there a family history of seizure activity?
   2. Assessment findings (see Table 2-5, p. 60)
   3. Diagnostic procedures
       a. Laboratory tests
           (1) Lumbar puncture (LP)—CSF abnormality caused by trauma or infection. Note: LP is not performed if increased ICP is suspected—a sudden decrease in pressure of CSF may result in herniation of the brain through the foramen magnum at the base of the skull.
           (2) CBC—increased WBC if infection present
           (3) Lead level—reveals increased levels, which may be cause of seizure
       b. Diagnostic studies
           (1) Electroencephalogram (EEG)—detects abnormal electrical activity and patterns specific to the seizure type
           (2) Computerized tomography (CT) scan—may reveal brain tumors, trauma, or infection as the cause of the seizure

F. **Therapeutic management**
   1. Medication
       a. Anticonvulsants—if active seizures, Ativan or Valium given; for maintenance, Dilantin, Phenobarbital commonly given by mouth
   2. Treatments

    a. Follow-up serum drug levels done particularly for evaluation of therapeutic levels of anticonvulsants

    b. Acute phase—oxygen therapy

G. Nursing management

  1. Acute care

    a. Nursing diagnosis: risk for injury

    b. Expected outcomes

      (1) Risk for injury will be reduced

      (2) Respiratory function will be maintained

    c. Interventions

      (1) Assess frequency, duration, and type of seizure activity

      (2) Observe for the following

        (a) Change in level of consciousness

        (b) Activity preceding seizure

        (c) Presence of aura—sensation experienced just before the onset of a seizure: sound, smell

        (d) Pupillary reaction postseizure

        (e) Incontinence of bowel, bladder, or both during or after seizure activity

        (f) LOC before and following seizure

      (3) Assess skin color, respiratory rate, signs of respiratory distress

      (4) Place in side-lying position with side rails up; remove sharp objects from bed; pad side rails; keep bed in low position

      (5) If not in bed during seizure, assist to floor; remove harmful objects; do not attempt to place objects in mouth or to restrain; loosen clothing; protect client from injury

      (6) Stay with client

      (7) Administer anticonvulsant as ordered

  2. Home care

    a. Nursing diagnosis: knowledge deficit

    b. Expected outcomes

      (1) Family will verbalize understanding of seizure disorder, treatment, and precautions

      (2) Therapeutic level of anticonvulsant will be maintained

    c. Interventions

      (1) Assess family's knowledge level regarding disorder, treatment, and seizure precautions

(2) Assess readiness for learning

(3) Discuss disease process and treatment

(4) Review medications and schedule for administration

(5) Review safety measures: medical alert tag; home safety

(6) Make referral to the Epilepsy Foundation

H. Evaluation

1. Questions to ask

   a. What are your concerns regarding long-term care?

   b. Do you have any questions about medication schedule, effects, or follow-up with physician?

2. Behaviors to observe

   a. Compliance with physician or clinic visits

   b. Statements regarding description of seizure and behaviors afterwards

   c. Reports signs of medication side effects

3. Evaluation of expected outcomes

   a. Injury is prevented

   b. Respiratory function is maintained

   c. Family states correct information regarding disorder, treatments, and medication regimen

   d. Therapeutic level of anticonvulsant is maintained

V. Head Trauma

A. **Description: An open or closed injury to cranium and its contents; includes concussions, contusions, skull fractures, cerebral edema, and vascular damage**

B. **Etiology and incidence**

   1. Injury is frequently due to mechanical force

   2. Falls are the leading cause of head injury; child abuse is the cause of severe head injury in children <1 year of age

   3. Adolescents most often receive head injuries in motor vehicle accidents

   4. Infants and toddlers are particularly vulnerable to head trauma because of proportionately large head size

   5. May be classified as localized or generalized

C. **Pathophysiology**

   1. Injury depends on force of impact

   2. Specific types of head injuries

      a. Concussion—a temporary and reversible neuronal dysfunction, characterized by posttraumatic amnesia

      b. Contusion and laceration—involves superficial tears and bruising of cerebral tissue, especially in occipital, temporal, and frontal lobes

      c. Fractures—linear, depressed, compound, basilar, and diastatic types

  3. Complications

      a. Epidural hemorrhage—arterial bleed

      b. Subdural hemorrhage—venous bleed

      c. Cerebral edema

      d. Postconcussion syndrome

D. Assessment

  1. Initial questions to ask

      a. What was the sequence of events for the trauma?

      b. Is there a history of a previous head injury?

  2. Assessment findings depend on severity (Box 2-3, p. 49)

  3. Diagnostic procedures

      a. Laboratory tests: none

      b. Diagnostic studies

          (1) Skull x-ray

          (2) Electroencephalogram (EEG)—reveals seizure activity

          (3) Computerized tomography (CT) scan—diagnoses neurological trauma

          (4) Magnetic resonance imaging (MRI)—detects intracranial injury

E. Therapeutic management

  1. Medications

      a. Antibiotics—if open injury is present

      b. Osmotic diuretics—if cerebral edema is present

      c. Anticonvulsant—for control of seizure activity

  2. Treatments

      a. Oxygen therapy

      b. Surgery—in the event of hemorrhage or skull fracture

F. Nursing management

  1. Acute care

      a. Nursing diagnosis: altered tissue perfusion—cerebral

      b. Expected outcomes: optimal cerebral perfusion is maintained

      c. Interventions

          (1) Assess neurological status every 1 to 2 hours: level of consciousness (LOC) (using Glasgow coma scale); orientation to time, place, person; pupil size

and reaction to light; speech patterns and thought processes

    (2) Monitor for signs of increased ICP

    (3) Monitor oxygen and CO_2 levels via arterial blood gases or pulse oximetry (O_2 saturation)

    (4) Monitor I&O

    (5) Assess child for pain or fever

    (6) Administer pain relief or osmotic diuretics as ordered

  d. Nursing diagnosis: risk for injury—seizures

  e. Expected outcome: additional injury from seizure activity is prevented

  f. Interventions: (refer to nursing care of child with seizures)

G. Evaluation

  1. Questions to ask

    a. What are your concerns about long-term care?

    b. What has the physician discussed regarding rehabilitation?

  2. Behaviors to observe

    a. Parents appropriately monitor and support child during and after seizure activity

    b. Family members ask questions regarding condition, treatment, outcome, and home care

  3. Evaluation of expected outcomes

    a. Prevention of injury from seizure activity achieved

    b. Maintenance of respiratory function with improved neurologic status attained

    c. Family members verbalize specific plans for rehabilitation, have contact with a head injury support group

Box 2-1. Signs of Increased Intracranial Pressure (ICP) in Infants and Children

Infants

Tense, bulging fontanel; lack of normal pulsations
Separated cranial sutures
Macewen sign—percussion of head elicits a cracked-pot sound
Irritability
High-pitched cry
Increased occipitofrontal circumference (OFC)
Distended scalp veins
Changes in feeding
Cries when held or rocked
"Setting sun" sign—eyes deviate with the iris downward to where a
  significant white part of the eye is found above the iris

Children

Headache
Nausea
Vomiting—often without nausea
Diplopia, blurred vision
Seizures

Personality and Behavior Signs

Irritability (toddlers), restlessness
Indifference, drowsiness, or lack of interest
Decline in school performance
Diminished physical activity and motor performance
Increased complaints of fatigue, tiredness; increased time devoted to sleep
Significant weight loss possible from anorexia and vomiting
Memory loss if pressure is greatly increased
Inability to follow simple commands
Progression to lethargy and drowsiness

Late Signs

Lowered level of consciousness
Decreased motor response to command
Decreased sensory response to painful stimuli
Alterations in pupil size and reactivity
Sometimes decerebrate or decorticate posturing
Cheyne-Stokes respirations
Papilledema

Box 2-2. Staging Criteria for Reye's Syndrome

Stage I   Vomiting, lethargy, and drowsiness; liver dysfunction; type I EEG, follows commands, pupillary reaction brisk

Stage II   Disorientation, combativeness, delirium, hyperventilation, hyperactive reflexes, appropriate responses to painful stimuli; evidence of liver dysfunction; type I EEG, pupillary reaction sluggish

Stage III   Obtunded, coma, hyperventilation, decorticate rigidity, preservation of pupillary light reaction and oculovestibular reflexes (although sluggish); type II EEG

Stage IV   Deepening coma, decerebrate rigidity, loss of oculocephalic reflexes, large and fixed pupils, loss of doll's eye reflex, loss of corneal reflexes; minimum liver dysfunction; type III or IV EEG, evidence of brain stem dysfunction

Stage V   Seizures, loss of deep tendon reflexes, respiratory arrest, flaccidity; type IV EEG; usually no evidence of liver dysfunction

Box 2-3. Clinical Manifestations of Acute Head Injury

Minor Injury

May or may not lose consciousness
Transient period of confusion
Somnolence
Listlessness
Irritability
Pallor
Vomiting (one or more episodes)

Signs of Progression

Altered mental status (e.g., difficulty rousing child)
Mounting agitation
Development of focal lateral neurologic signs
Marked changes in vital signs

Severe Injury

Signs of increased ICP (see Box 8-1 p. 199)
    Increased head size (infant)
    Bulging fontanel (infant)
Retinal hemorrhage
Extraocular palsies (especially cranial nerve VI)
Hemiparesis
Quadriplegia
Elevated temperature (sometimes)
Unsteady gait (older child)
Papilledema (older child)

Associated Signs

Skin injury (to area of head sustaining injury)
Other injuries (e.g., to extremities)

Table 2-1. Structure and Function of the Brain

Structure	Function	Effects of Dysfunction
Cerebrum	Consciousness, thought process, memory Sensory input Motor activity	Dependent on specific site involved
▼ Frontal lobes	Motor activity Social Interaction Abstract thinking Expressive language	Anterior damage—personality changes Memory defects Language defects
▼ Parietal lobes	Sensation Smaller interpretation	Language dysfunction Lower motor and sensory loss Aphasia
Cerebellum	Muscle movement: coordination and refinement	Ataxia Nystagmus Dystonia
Basal Ganglia	Automatic control of lower motor centers	Athetosis Tremors at rest nonintention'
Diencephalon	Forms reticular activating system	Stupor
▼ Thalamus	Sensory impulse relay station to cerebral cortex	Altered consciousness
▼ Hypothalamus	Control center for involuntary activities ▼ Blood pressure ▼ Satiety ▼ Hunger ▼ Temperature regulation ▼ Sleep regulation	Coma Weight loss, anorexia Endocrine disorders

Table 2-1. Structure and Function of the Brain—cont'd

Structure	Function	Effects of Dysfunction
Brain stem	Gives rise to cranial nerves	Stupor, coma
▼ Midbrain	Connection between hindbrain and forebrain Holds nuclei for cranial nerves III, IV, part of V	Altered consciousness Decerebrate posturing Neurologic hyperventilation
▼ Pons	Respiratory center (pneumotaxic center) Cranial nerves V through VIII	Deep, rapid, or periodic breathing Impaired cranial nerve function (V through VIII)
▼ Medulla	Respiratory center Cranial nerves IX, X, XI, XII	Biot's respiration Flaccid muscle tone Absence of deep tendon, gag and corneal reflexes

Modified from Wong, D: *Whaley and Wong's nursing care of infants and children,* ed 5, St Louis, 1995, Mosby.

Table 2-2. Levels of Consciousness

State	Description and Characteristics
Sleep (normal unconsciousness)	Cyclic (regularly recurring) physiologic state Reversible by auditory, visual, or tactile stimuli Immobile posture Absence of alertness, cognition, voluntary movement Body processes partially suspended Intermittent dreaming; may be able to recall dream
Confusion	Fails to comprehend surroundings Appears to lose proper bearings Unable to estimate direction or location Likely to be disoriented in time May misidentify people Short attention span, difficulty in following even simple directions Tends to misinterpret events May be hyperactive or apathetic and immobile Usually able to give relevant answers to simple questions about age or location of pain Gives irrelevant and inaccurate answers to more complex questions Alert; arousal responses intact
Delirium	Confusion, disorientation, fear, irritability, agitation, hyperactivity Illusions—false interpretation of sensory perceptions Hallucinations—false sensory perceptions Delusions—false ideas Typically loud, talkative, suspicious, agitated Often associated with high fever, toxic substances, shock states Tremulousness, sweating Frequently responds with a "startle" reaction to unexpected stimuli

Table 2-2. Levels of Consciousness—cont'd

State	Description and Characteristics
Pseudowakeful states (akinetic mutism, apallic syndrome)	Sits or lies with eyes open but fails to follow objects or lights Does not turn eyes toward a noise Does not speak May follow objects or persons with eyes, may turn slowly toward a sound and appear about to speak, but remains silent (reptilian stare) Response to external stimuli similar to that of stupor or light coma May be restless and hyperkinetic May remain motionless and speechless
Comatose states	Diminished alertness Occurs as a continuum Extends from somnolence to deep coma

Modified from Wong, D: *Whaley and Wong's nursing care of infants and children,* ed 5, St Louis, 1995, Mosby.

Table 2-3. Major Neurologic Diagnostic Procedures

Procedure	Purpose	Indication	Developmental Considerations
Lumbar puncture (LP)	To obtain CSF for visualization, laboratory analysis, and pressure reading To inject medication or spinal anesthesia	Meningitis, encephalitis CNS hemorrhage	Child, toddler, or infant placed in side-lying position with knees and head flexed (fetal-like position)
Subdural tap	To remove accumulation of fluid from subdural hematomas, cerebral effusion	Subdural hematoma, cerebral effusion	Infant may be wrapped in mummy restraint Infant must be placed in infant seat or semi-upright position following tap. Older children may benefit from therapeutic play
Radiography	Reveals fractures, dislocations, spreading suture lines Reveals degenerative changes	Trauma of skull, spinal column Headaches Congenital malformation	Noninvasive; machinery may be frightening and cold Parent may need to accompany child

Test	Description	Indications	Nursing considerations
Computed tomography (CT scan)	Horizontal and vertical cross section of brain may be visualized Indicates tissue density	Neurologic trauma Unconsciousness Hydrocephalus Lesions, tumors	Sedation usually necessary, since child needs to remain still An infant may be fed 30 minutes before test to facilitate sleep Child NPO before procedure
Electroencephalography (EEG)	Measures electrical activity of cerebral cortex	Determination of brain death Diagnosis of seizures Sleep abnormalities	Minimize external stimuli Child must lie quietly during 45 minute procedure
Magnetic Resonance Imaging (MRI)	Evaluates soft tissue of brain and spinal column	Tumors, hemorrhages Vascular disorders Congenital malformations	Sedation may be required Parent may remain with child to provide reassurance

Modified from Wong, D: *Whaley and Wong's nursing care of infants and children*, ed 5, St Louis, 1995, Mosby.

Table 2-4. Common Medications for CNS Disorders

Classification	Medication	Indications	Route and Dosage	Side Effects	Nursing Implications
Anticonvulsant	Generic: phenobarb Trade: Luminal	All types of seizures except absence Reye's syndrome	PO (seizures) 3-5 mg/kg/day IV (status epilepticus) 15-18 mg/kg over 10-15 min. Maintenance: (may divide doses) *Infants:* 5-6 mg/kg/day *1-5 years old:* 6-8 mg/kg/day *6-12 years old:* 4-6 mg/kg/day *>12 years old:* 1-3 mg/kg/day	*CNS:* Drowsiness, ataxia, irritability, headache *GI:* Nausea, vomiting *Hepatic:* Jaundice, hepatitis *GU:* Renal damage *Integumentary:* Rash, dermatitis *Hematology:* Bone marrow suppression *Metabolic:* Hypocalcemia *Respiratory:* Respiratory depression	Assess level of consciousness Assess respiratory status Medication may be mixed with food Monitor vital signs, CBC, liver and renal function studies when on long-term therapy *Parent education:* Do not discontinue drug or increase dosage Do not administer with other drugs or ETOH May affect cognitive learning
Anticonvulsant	Generic: lorazapam Trade: Ativan	Status Epilepticus	IV 0.05-0.2 mg/kg over 2 minutes	*CNS:* Dizziness, drowsiness *CV:* Orthostatic hypotension, tachycardia	Preferred drug, since it has longer duration and causes less respiratory distress than Valium

| Anticonvulsant | Generic: phenytoin Trade: Dilantin | Used for tonic-clonic and partial seizures, status epilepticus | PO 5 mg/kg in 2-3 doses and adjusted IV (status epilepticus) 10-15 mg/kg/day *6 mo-3 yr:* 8-10 mg/kg/day in 2 or 3 divided doses *4 yr-6 yr:* 7.5-9 mg/kg/day in 2 or 3 divided doses *10-16 yr:* 6-7 mg/kg/day in 2 or 3 divided doses | *CNS:* Confusion, dizziness, drowsiness, insomnia *CV:* Bradycardia, hypotension, cardiac arrest *EENT:* Gingival hypertrophy, slurred speech *GI:* Nausea, vomiting anorexia, diarrhea, weight loss *Integumentary:* Hirsutism, rash, dermatitis *Hematology:* Neutropenia | Assess Dilantin level (therapeutic level, 10-20 mg/ml) Stress patient compliance to prevent seizure activity Administer with food to decrease GI upset Stress importance of dental hygiene; gingival hypertrophy is side effect— enlarged, sensitive gums Monitor blood, liver, and renal studies in long-term therapy Advise patient that urine may turn pink to brown in color |

Continued.

Table 2-4. Common Medications for CNS Disorders—cont'd

Classification	Medication	Indications	Route and Dosage	Side Effects	Nursing Implications
Antibiotic	Generic: methicillin Trade: Staphcillin	Bacterial meningitis caused by staphylococcus Hydrocephalus shunt infection	IM, IV Children: 100-400 mg/kg/day q 4-6 hr in equally divided doses	*GI:* Hairy tongue, oral lesions *GU:* Intestinal nephritis *Integumentary:* Urticarial rash *Hematology:* Esinophilia, anemia, neuropenia *Other:* Hypersensitivity	Assess for previous allergies to methicillin, penicillins, cephalosporins Assess baseline blood, renal, and hepatic tests Maintain adequate hydration to prevent hemorrhagic cystitis Monitor IV site for vein irritation and thrombophlibitis
Antibiotic, third-generation cephalosporin	Generic: ceftriaxone sodium Trade: Rocephin	Infections caused by gram-negative and some gram-positive bacteria Meningitis	IM, IV *Infant and child infections:* 50-75 mg/kg/day q 12 hr in equally divided doses, not to exceed 2 g/day *Meningitis:* 100 mg/kg/day in two divided doses; not to exceed 4 g/day	*CNS:* Headache, dizziness *GI:* Nausea, vomiting, diarrhea, pseudo membranous colitis *GU:* Vaginitis, proteinuria *Hematology:* Leukopenia, anemia, thrombocytopenia *Integumentary:* Rash, pruritis *Respiratory:* Dyspnea	Assess previous allergy to penicillins or other cephalosporins Assess for allergic reactions Monitor for signs of superinfection Recommend daily yogurt to maintain normal intestinal flora

Diuretic; carbonic anhydrous inhibitor	Generic: acetazolamide Trade: Diamox	Decreased CSF production in hydro-cephalus	PO 8-30 mg/kg/day in four divided doses IV, IM 5-10 mg/kg/day	*CNS*: Drowsiness, anxiety, depression *EENT*: Myopia, tinnitus *GI*: Nausea, vomiting, metallic taste *GU*: Frequency, hypokalemia, polyuria *Hematology*: Leukopenia *Integumentary*: Rash, pruritis, urticaria	Monitor daily weights, I&O Administer potassium supplement as ordered Recommend high-potassium foods in diet *Parent education*: Advise family to report sore throat, bruising, or bleeding Avoid activities that require alertness Child should wear sunscreen
Osmotic diuretic	Generic: mannitol Trade: Osmitrol	Cerebral edema Intraocular pressure increased Induce diuresis in Reye's Syndrome	IV 1-2 g/kg	*CNS*: Headache, dizziness *CV*: Hypotension, tachycardia *GI*: Nausea, vomiting *GU*: Electrolyte imbalance *Integumentary*: Rash, hives	Assess serum electrolytes and vital signs with BP lying and standing Daily weights Assess for respiratory status and changes in heart rate

Table 2-5. Types of Seizures

Seizure Type	Assessment Findings	Age of Onset	Frequency	Loss of Consciousness
Partial				
▶ Simple partial	Unilateral localized motor and sensory impairment Twitching, tingling, numbness	Any age	Variable	No
▶ Complex partial	Staring Lip smacking, eye blinking Chewing Purposeless behaviors	Age 3 and over	1-2 times/day	Mental disorientation Impaired consciousness
Generalized				
▶ Absence	Minor muscle twitching	Age 3 and over	Multiple/day	Brief loss of awareness
▶ Tonic-clonic	Rolling eyes upward Falls to ground Arms flex; legs, head, and neck extend Muscles rhythmically contract and relax	Childhood (typically from temperatures >102° F)	Variable	Yes

Modified from Betz and Poster, *Mosby's pediatric nursing reference*, ed 2, St Louis, 1992, Mosby.

REVIEW QUESTIONS

1. An infant is scheduled for surgery to repair myelomeningocele. Preoperatively, which of these nursing diagnoses should receive priority in the infant's care?
   a. Altered family processes
   b. Risk for infection
   c. Knowledge deficit
   d. Altered growth and development

2. A child exhibits seizure activity. Which of these actions should the nurse take?
   a. Attempt to restrain the child
   b. Insert a padded tongue blade into the mouth
   c. Prevent the child from hitting hard or sharp objects
   d. Suction mouth as needed to maintain the airway

3. An infant's diagnosis is myelomeningocele. To protect the sac from infection, which of these actions is appropriate?
   a. Change diapers as soon as they are soiled
   b. Apply sterile, dry dressings to sac
   c. Elevate head of crib to high fowler's position
   d. Place infant in supine position at all times

4. Immediately following insertion of a ventriculoperitoneal shunt, the nurse should expect to position the infant
   a. On the operative side with the head of crib elevated
   b. On the nonoperative side with the crib flat
   c. Supine with the head of the crib elevated
   d. Supine with the crib flat

5. A child diagnosed with meningitis is restless and irritable when first hospitalized. To promote the child's comfort, which of these actions should the nurse take initially?
   a. Discourage parent from staying with child
   b. Keep environmental noise to a minimum
   c. Position the child in a supine position for 12 hours
   d. Postpone all scheduled testing

6. A child is admitted to the pediatric unit for seizure activity. The physician orders phenobarbital. The nurse provides the parents with instructions regarding the correct administration of this medication. The nurse would evaluate the teaching as effective when the parents identify the need to
   a. Skip a dose if the child vomits

    b. Discontinue the medication when seizure activity stops

    c. Double the next dose if the child misses a dose

    d. Notify the physician if severe headaches and skin rash occur

7. Before discharge, the parents have been given instructions regarding signs of a blocked shunt. Which of these statements by the parents indicates a correct understanding of home care parameters?

    a. "We'll notify the physician if we observe irritability and a bulging soft spot."

    b. "We'll notify the physician if the baby's temperature is 99 degrees."

    c. "Urine retention and cool skin are signs of a blocked shunt."

    d. "Vomiting and diarrhea are signs of a blocked shunt."

8. An infant is diagnosed with pneumococcal meningitis. The parents question the mode of transmission for this infectious agent. The nurse reviews the child's history. Which of the following should be considered?

    a. Chicken pox

    b. Middle ear infection

    c. Lyme disease

    d. Urinary tract infection

9. When performing a postoperative assessment on an infant with surgical correction of a myelomeningocele, the nurse observes bulging anterior fontanel and increased head size. Based on these findings the nurse knows the infant is at imminent risk for developing

    a. Encephalitis

    b. Hydrocephalus

    c. Meningitis

    d. Fluid overload

10. Considering the client's diagnosis of myelomeningocele, the infant is most likely to have which of these findings?

    a. Dyspnea and cardiac abnormalities

    b. Fecal continence and microcephalus

    c. Genitourinary and orthopedic abnormalities

    d. Meningeal sac everted and located in the thoracic region

11. Following surgical correction of myelomeningocele, which of these actions should receive priority?

    a. Place infant in prone or side-lying position

    b. Maintain hips in slight adduction

    c. Measure abdominal girth daily

    d. Weigh infant daily

ANSWERS, RATIONALES, AND TEST-TAKING TIPS

Rationales	Test-Taking Tips

1. Correct answer: b

Many myelomeningocele sacs are at risk for rupture during the delivery or the transport; any opening increases risk for infection. Although it is important for parents to understand the nature of a spinal defect and its impact on the child's growth, development, and family life, the immediate preoperative priority is prevention of infection.

The use of Maslow's hierarchy of needs can be applied here—the physiological needs are the first priority. Response *b* is a physiological need, whereas response *d* is both physical and psychological. Response *b* is the best answer.

2. Correct answer: c

The child, as any client, must be protected from injury during the seizure. The convulsing client should not be moved or restrained during a seizure. Force should not be exerted in an attempt to place solid objects between the teeth or to suction for airway maintenance.

Recall and associate *seizures* need *safety* as a priority.

3. Correct answer: a

The myelomeningocele sac must remain free of urine or stool contamination; therefore, frequent diaper changes are essential. Dressings applied to sac are to be moistened, usually with sterile normal saline, to prevent drying of the sac. Ideally, the infant in a prone or partially prone-to-side-lying position is placed

Eliminate response *b*, which has the word "dry," making it incorrect. Eliminate response *c*, which has "high fowler's" for a crib position; use common sense—if this was done the infant would slide down to the flat part of the crib. Eliminate response *d*, since it has the absolute "at all times," which means no other position can be used.

in a low Trendelenburg position to reduce spinal fluid pressure in the sac, with hips flexed to avoid pressure on the defect. Range of motion may need to be done to prevent flexion contractures.

4. Correct answer: b

Following this type of surgery, the infant is positioned on the nonoperative side to prevent pressure on the shunt valve and the pressure areas of the operative side. The crib is kept flat to prevent complications from a rapid reduction of intracranial fluid. Placed on the operative side, there is increased pressure on the shunt valve and the elevated head of the bed causes a rapid decrease in intracranial pressure. The items in options *c* and *d* are incorrect responses.

Remember a basic principle of postoperative care for clients with cranial and eye surgery: position the client on the nonoperative side for the prevention of increased pressure in the surgical area.

5. Correct answer: b

The room should be kept as quiet as possible and the environmental stimuli kept to a minimum, since most children are sensitive to noise, bright lights, and other environmental stimuli. The parents should be encouraged to stay with the child and become involve in the child's care to decrease separation anxiety. Usually

Eliminate responses *a* and *d* with the use of common sense—test postponement is usually wrong, as is not having the parents present. Response *c* is incorrect— the child won't be able to assume a comfortable supine position, and special positioning for 12 hours has nothing to do with this type of problem.

the child assumes a side-lying position because of nuchal rigidity and the tendency to hyperextension of the neck. Acute meningitis is a medical emergency. Early recognition of causative organisms through testing is essential. Expedient therapy with medication prevents death and disability.

6. Correct answer: d

Parents need to know the adverse reactions to the seizure medication phenobarb. Severe headaches and skin rash are side effects that need to be reported. The other responses reflect a need for more education. The family should be taught the necessity of continuing the medication regularly without interruption, not doubling the dose, and notifying the health professional when the child has an illness, including vomiting.

If you have no idea of the correct answer, try clustering under inappropriate medication guidelines. Key words concerning the medication dose in responses *a, b,* and *c* are: "skip," "discontinue," and "double."

7. Correct answer: a

Parents need to recognize signs that indicate shunt malfunction; these include irritability and bulging fontanel, which are signs of increased intracranial pressure. A 99 degree temperature is not significant to warrant notification of physician. The findings in options *c* and *d* are not specific

Associate "blocked shunt" with the result of increased pressure—select response *a*, which has the key words "irritability" and "bulging . . . spot."

to a blocked shunt. Vomiting by itself, especially projectile, would indicate increased intracranial pressure and should be reported.

8. **Correct answer: b**

   Meningitis and other suppurative intracranial complications are common extensions of an infection from the middle ear or mastoid. Middle ear infections are frequently bacterial infections.

   Chicken pox is caused by varicella virus. Lyme disease is caused by a spirochete, which enters the skin through a tick bite. The majority of urinary tract infections are caused by E. coli and other gram-negative organisms common to anal, perineal, and perianal regions. If you have no idea of the correct response, try the common sense approach associated with anatomical location. Select the given area that is closest to the brain—response *b,* the middle ear.

9. **Correct answer: b**

   The anomaly most frequently associated with myelomeningocele is hydrocephalus—an obstruction to CSF caused by downward displacement of brain stem and cerebellum through the foramen magnum. A bulging fontanel and increased head size are consistent with increased intracranial pressure caused by the blockage of CSF. In options *a, c,* and *d* the findings are not consistent with encephalitis or fluid overload. Bacterial meningitis is a complication of otitis media.

   Note that responses *a* and *c* contain *-itis* which suggests inflammation; this is not a typically a postoperative problem. Select response *b* rather than response *d,* since fluid overload is more often indicated by abnormal pulmonary or cardiac findings.

10. Correct answer: c

Myelomeningocele is one of the most common causes of neurogenic bladder. Orthopedic anomalies of the hip, knee, and foot are possible depending on location of the spinal lesion. The findings in option *a* are not consistent with a neural tube defect. Fecal incontinence and hydrocephalus are most often evident in myelomeningocele. The largest number of these defects are located in the lumbar or lumbosacral region.

Note that if response *b* was read quickly, you may have misread "continence" as "incontinence" and selected it as even though microcephalus is not found.

11. Correct answer: a

A prone position is maintained postoperatively, although a side-lying or partial side-lying position may also be used unless hip dysplasia is present. These side-lying positions allow for positional changes, which decrease the risk of pressure sores and eases efforts to feed. The legs are maintained in abduction with a pad between the knees to counteract hip subluxation. The action in option *c* is not appropriate. Weighing the infant is a general action of any postsurgical infant's plan of care.

If you narrowed the responses to *a* and *d,* reread the question and note that the question is for the *priority.* Since the surgery is on the nervous system, positioning takes precedent over weights, which would be done routinely on infants and children.

Nursing Care of Children with Cardiovascular Disorders

STUDY OUTCOMES

After completing this chapter, the reader will be able to do the following:

▼ State circulatory changes that occur at birth.

▼ Describe nursing priorities for the child in congestive heart failure.

▼ Verbalize a description of altered hemodynamics associated with congenital defects.

▼ Describe a plan of care for the child with an acyanotic cardiac defect.

▼ State four defects associated with Tetralogy of Fallot.

▼ Outline a plan of care for the child with a cyanotic defect.

▼ Describe priorities in the management of the child with rheumatic fever.

KEY TERMS

Afterload	Resistance against which the left or right ventricle must eject its volume of blood during contraction; resistance is produced by the volume of blood already in the vascular system and the vessel walls: for the right ventricle the pulmonary vascular system (called pulmonary vascular resistance, PVR) and for the left ventricle the systemic vascular system (called systemic vascular resistance, SVR).
Hypoxemia	Abnormal deficiency of oxygen in the arterial system; chronic hypoxemia stimulates red blood cell production leading to secondary polycythemia; if caused by decreased alveolar oxygen tension or underventilation, improvement occurs with oxygen administration; if caused by shunting of blood from right to left heart without exchange of gases in the lungs, improvement is achieved by bronchial hygiene and positive end expiratory pressure therapy.
Hypoxia	Inadequate oxygen at the cellular level; tissues most sensitive hypoxia are the brain, heart, pulmonary vessels, and liver.
Hypoxic drive	Low arterial oxygen pressure stimulus to respiration that is mediated through the carotid and aortic bodies, also called chemoreceptors for $PaCO_2$.
Preload	Stretch of the myocardial fiber at end diastole, which is reflected by the ventricular end diastolic pressure and volume.

CONTENT REVIEW

I. Cardiovascular (CV) system overview

   A. **General concepts**
      1. Heart lies in the thoracic cavity; in infants and children the heart lies more horizontally in the chest
      2. Apex of the heart extends into the fourth left intercostal space (ICS) until 7 years of age
      3. Fetal oxygenation of blood occurs in the placenta
   B. **Review of heart structure and function**
      1. Structure

    a. Pericardium—tough, double-walled sac that protects heart

    b. Three layers of heart wall

       (1) Epicardium—thin, outermost layer covering surface of heart

       (2) Myocardium—middle layer of heart wall responsible for pumping action of ventricles; consists of striated muscle fibers

       (3) Endocardium—innermost layer; lines inner chambers of heart and covers heart valves

    b. Four chambers

       (1) Right and left atria—act as reservoirs for blood returning from the veins

       (2) Right and left ventricles—pump blood to the lungs (right) and throughout the body (left)

    c. Left and right sides of heart are divided by the cardiac septum

       (1) Left heart consists of left atrium, left ventricle, and aorta

       (2) Right heart consists of right atrium, right ventricle, and pulmonary artery

    d. Two sets of valves

       (1) Atrioventricular—tricuspid and mitral

       (2) Semilunar—pulmonic and aortic

    e. Pressure differences between the right and left side of heart (blood flows from area of greatest pressure to area of least pressure), regulates the flow of blood through heart and into systemic circulation (Figure 3-1)

    f. Great vessels—arteries and veins located in cluster at base of heart

       (1) Aorta—carries oxygenated blood out from the left ventricle to the body

       (2) Superior and inferior vena cavae—carry unoxygenated blood from upper and lower body, respectively, to right atrium

       (3) Pulmonary artery—leaves right ventricle, branches, and carries unoxygenated blood to lungs

       (4) Pulmonary vein—returns oxygenated blood from lungs to left atrium

2. Function and development

    a. Primary purpose of the CV system is to pump oxygen and nutrients throughout the body and remove the end products of metabolism

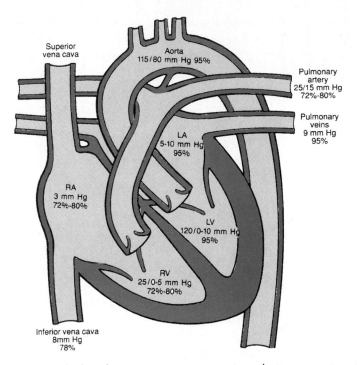

Figure 3-1. Normal chamber pressure (mm Hg) and O_2 saturation (SaO$_2$) in cardiac chambers and great vessels. (From Wong, D: *Whaley and Wong's nursing care of infants and children*, ed 5, St Louis, 1995, Mosby.)

    b. The heart develops between the fourth and eighth weeks of gestation

    c. Fetal vascular resistance is high

    d. Fetal structures provide for a pattern of intrauterine circulation

        (1) Foramen ovale—pumps blood from right to left atrium

        (2) Ductus arteriosus—shunts blood from pulmonary artery to the descending aorta

        (3) Ductus venosus—shunts most of blood supply around the fetal liver

    e. Circulatory changes that result in postnatal circulation (Figure 3-2)

        (1) Dilatation of the pulmonary vessels and decreased pulmonary vascular resistance as the lungs expand at birth

        (2) A rise in systemic vascular resistance, which causes increased pressure in left side of heart when umbilical cord is clamped

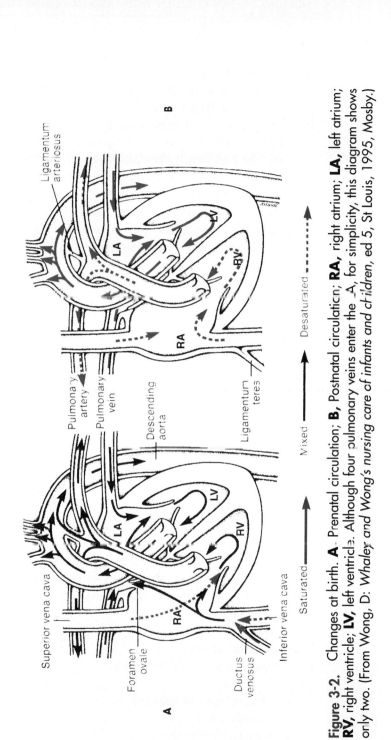

Figure 3-2. Changes at birth. **A,** Prenatal circulation; **B,** Postnatal circulation; **RA,** right atrium; **LA,** left atrium; **RV,** right ventricle; **LV,** left ventricle. Although four pulmonary veins enter the _A, for simplicity, this diagram shows only two. (From Wong, D: Whaley and Wong's nursing care of infants and children, ed 5, St Louis, 1995, Mosby.)

          (3) Closure of the foramen ovale usually occurs shortly after birth

          (4) Closure of the ductus arteriosus usually occurs by the fourth day of life

   3. Basic concepts of cardiac physiology

      a. To provide effective oxygen transport to the tissues of the body, the heart must maintain adequate cardiac output (CO) pumped per unit of time: CO equals stroke volume × heart rate: $CO = SV \times HR$

      b. Stroke volume is the amount of blood ejected by the heart during any one contraction; it is influenced by

          (1) Preload—the volume or fiber length of the ventricles before contraction

          (2) Afterload—the resistance that the ventricles encounter during contraction

          (3) Contractility—the ability of the heart muscle to act as an efficient pump through myocardial fiber shortening

II. Assessment

  A. Health history

    1. Questions to ask

      a. Activity

          (1) Does the infant tire easily during feeding?

          (2) Does the child tire easily during play?

          (3) Does the child perspire during activity?

          (4) Does the child have frequent infections?

          (5) Does the child nap longer than expected?

          (6) Does the child squat rather than sit when at play?

          (7) Does the child turn blue during crying episodes?

          (8) Does the child experience leg pains while running?

      b. Diet/nutrition: Is the child's weight gain as expected?

    2. Present problem

      a. Fatigue

      b. Leg pain or cramps

      c. Frequent respiratory infections

    3. History

      a. Cardiac surgery or evaluation

      b. Rheumatic fever

      c. Congenital cardiac defect

      d. Mother's health during pregnancy: rubella or other infections in the first trimester; drug or alcohol use

    e. Apgar score, gestational age, complications at birth

    f. Down syndrome

  4. Family history

    a. Heart disease

    b. Hyperlipidemia

    c. Congenital heart defects

    d. Hypertension

B. Physical examination

  1. Sequence

    a. Observation of general appearance

      (1) Positioning

      (2) Respirations

      (3) Skin color

      (4) Nail color and configuration

    b. Assessment and palpation of the anterior chest precordium

    c. Carotid artery palpation

    d. Blood pressure assessment: compare readings obtained from upper and lower extremities

    e. Auscultation of the following areas for rate, rhythm, pitch, location, and intensity of S_1 and S_2 (Figure 3-3)

      (1) Aortic area

      (2) Pulmonic area

      (3) Third left intercostal space

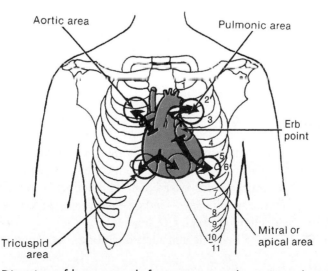

Figure 3-3. Direction of heart sounds for anatomic valve sites and areas (circled) for auscultation. (From Wong, D: *Whaley and Wong's nursing care of infants and children,* ed 5, St Louis, 1995, Mosby.)

            (4) Tricuspid area

            (5) Apical area—will be at 4 ICS until 7 years of age

      f. Auscultation of murmurs, pericardial rubs, extra heart sounds—S_3,S_4

  2. Pediatric considerations

      a. Venous hum heard at medial end of clavicle and interior border of sternocleidomastoid muscle, is usually insignificant

      b. Rheumatic fever accounts for most acquired murmurs in children

      c. Sinus dysrhythmias are considered normal in children

      d. Priorities when examining a child with known heart disease

            (1) Weight gain

            (2) Edema—periorbital, peripheral

            (3) Respiratory status—tachypnea

            (4) Developmental delay

            (5) Cyanosis—central, peripheral

            (6) Enlarged neck veins

            (7) Clubbing of fingers and toes

            (8) Murmurs, bruits, and thrills

      e. Selecting the correct size of blood pressure cuff is essential: cuff width should cover approximately two thirds of the upper arm

C. Diagnostic and laboratory tests

  1. Cardiac catheterization—reveals abnormal communication between chambers of the heart, as well as pressure differences and abnormal blood gas sampling in the chambers; helps in location of a septal defect

  2. Electrocardiography (ECG)—reveals atrial and ventricular hypertrophy, as well as dysrhythmias

  3. Echocardiography—reveals changes in valve function, great vessel location and size, presence of shunting within the heart

  4. CBC

      a. Indicates increased HCT (polycythemia), Hgb, and erythrocytes possibly from chronic hypoxia

      b. Indicates decreased platelet function, thrombocytopenia

  5. Arterial blood gases—indicate degree of acid-base balance; O_2 saturation; O_2 level; CO_2 level

  6. PT, A PTT—indicates altered clotting mechanism if increased

III. Medications

  A. Priority drug classifications

    1. Cardiac glycosides

    2. Diuretics
    3. Antiarrhythmics
    4. Antibiotics
  B. Refer to Table 3-1, pp. 100-105

IV. Acyanotic heart defects

  A. Definition: congenital abnormalities of the heart in which mainly oxygenated blood enters systemic circulation

  B. Acyanotic defects, according to the hemodynamic classification system

    1. Increased pulmonary blood flow
      a. Atrial septal defect (ASD)
      b. Ventricular septal defect (VSD)
      c. Patent ductus arteriosus (PDA)
      d. Endocardial cushion defect (ECD)
    2. Obstruction to blood flow *from* ventricles
      a. Coarctation of aorta
      b. Aortic stenosis (AS)
      c. Pulmonic stenosis (PS)

  C. Etiology and incidence

    1. Mostly unknown; prenatal factors include
      a. Teratogenic exposure during first trimester of pregnancy: rubella, drugs, alcohol
      b. Maternal type 1 diabetes
      c. Maternal age >40 years
    2. Genetic factors are also implicated
    3. Most common acynotic defect: ventricular septal defect (VSD) accounts for 30% of all defects

  D. Pathophysiology

    1. ASD
      a. Abnormal opening in the septum that separates the right and left atria; defect may be one of three types
        (1) Ostium primum: defect located at lower end of the septum
        (2) Ostium secundum: defect at the center of the septum
        (3) Sinus venosus: defect at the junction of the superior vena cava and the right atrium
      b. Oxygenated blood flows through the opening from an area of higher pressure (left atria) to an area of lower pressure (right atria) (Figure 3-4)
      c. Increased compliance of the right atrium and right ventricle causes an increased volume of blood flow into the lungs

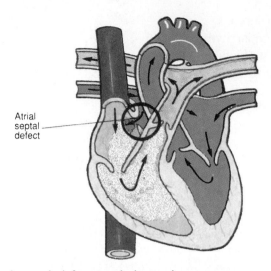

Atrial
septal
defect

Figure 3-4. Atrial septal defect (circled). Darker areas, saturated blood; lighter blue areas, mixed blood; gray areas, desaturated blood. (From Wong, D: *Whaley and Wong's nursing care of infants and children,* ed 5, St Louis, 1995, Mosby.)

2. Endocardial cushion defect or atrioventricular canal defect
   a. Results from an incomplete closure of the endocardial cushion; severity of the defect varies
   b. Abnormalities occur in the septa of the atria and the ventricles and in the atrioventricular valve(s) (Figure 3-5)
   c. Pulmonary vascular engorgement occurs with left-to-right shunting
3. VSD
   a. Abnormal opening in the septum that separates the right and left ventricles
   b. This opening allows oxygenated blood to flow from the left to the right ventricle (Figure 3-6)
   c. Increased blood to the pulmonary circulation results in frequent respiratory infections, increased pulmonary vascular resistance (PVR), right-sided enlargement of heart, and congestive heart failure (CHF)
4. PDA
   a. Abnormal passageway between the aortic and the pulmonary circulation that occurs when the ductus arteriosus fails to close after birth
   b. Left-to-right shunting of oxygenated blood is recirculated through the lungs, to the left atrium, and the left ventricle

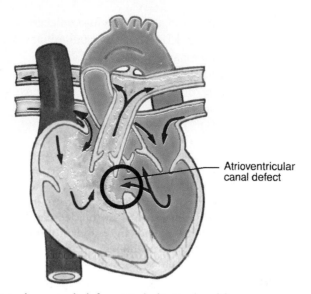

Figure 3-5. Atrioventricular canal defect (circled). Darker blue areas, saturated blood; gray areas, desaturated blood; lighter blue areas, mixed blood. (From Wong, D: *Whaley and Wong's nursing care of infants and children,* ed 5, St Louis, 1995, Mosby.)

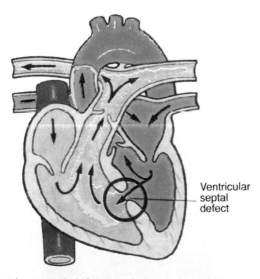

Figure 3-6. Ventricular septal defect (circled). Darker blue areas, saturated blood; gray areas, desaturated blood; light blue areas, mixed blood. (From Wong, D: *Whaley and Wong's nursing care of infants and children,* ed 5, St Louis, 1995, Mosby.)

      c. Left atrial and ventricular enlargement occur as a result of a large PDA; increased pulmonary pressure leads to pulmonary edema and CHF

  5. Coarctation of aorta

      a. Narrowing of aortic lumen; the position of defect is classified as

          (1) Juxtaductal—at the level of the ductus arteriosus

          (2) Preductal—proximal to the ductus arteriosus

          (3) Postductal—distal to the ductus arteriosus (Figure 3-7)

      b. Results in decreased blood flow distal to the defect and increased pressure proximal to the defect

      c. Associated with other defects, such as bicuspid aortic valve and VSD

  6. Aortic stenosis

      a. Narrowing of the aortic valve that results in resistance to left ventricular ejection of blood (Figure 3-8)

      b. The left ventricle hypertrophies from the increased workload

      c. Pulmonary edema occurs from left ventricular failure and increased left atrial pressures

  7. Pulmonic stenosis

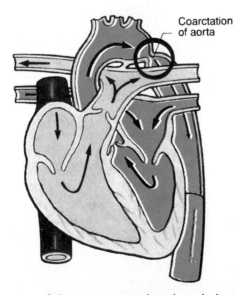

Figure 3-7. Coarctation of the Aorta (postductal circled). Blue areas, saturated blood; gray areas, desaturated blood. (From Wong, D: *Whaley and Wong's nursing care of infants and children*, ed 5, St Louis, 1995, Mosby.)

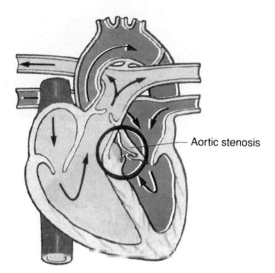

Figure 3-8. Aortic stenosis (circled). Blue areas, saturated blood; darker gray areas, desaturated blood. (From Wong, D: *Whaley and Wong's nursing care of infants and children,* ed 5, St Louis, 1995, Mosby.)

       a. Narrowing of one or more sites at the entrance to the pulmonary artery

       b. Right ventricular hypertrophy occurs with resistance to blood flow (Figure 3-9)

       c. Right ventricular failure may eventually occur and force reopening of the foramen ovale and the shunting of unoxygenated blood into the systemic circulation

E. Assessment (Table 3-2, p. 106)

F. Therapeutic management

    1. Medications

       a. Diuretics: chlorothiazide (Diuril), spironolactone (Aldactone), furosemide (Lasix)

       b. Cardiac glycosides: digoxin (Lanoxin)

       c. Electrolyte replacement: potassium (Klorvess)

       d. Bronchodilators: beta adrenergic stimulant—isoproterenol (Isuprel): increases cardiac output; dilates bronchioles

    2. Treatment: conservative until surgery

    3. Surgery: refer to Table 3-2, p. 106, for surgical procedures performed for various defects

G. Nursing management: child with an acyanotic defect

    1. Acute care: presurgical

       a. Nursing diagnosis: decreased cardiac output

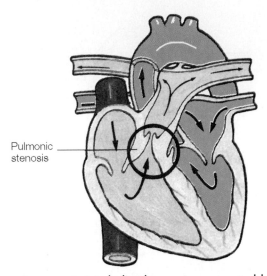

Pulmonic
stenosis

Figure 3-9. Pulmonic stenosis (circled). Blue areas, saturated blood; darker gray areas, desaturated blood. (From Wong, D: *Whaley and Wong's nursing care of infants and children,* ed 5, St Louis, 1995, Mosby.)

      b. Expected outcomes
          (1) Return to or maintain stable vital signs
          (2) Child will maintain adequate tissue perfusion as evidenced by normal color
      c. Interventions
          (1) Assess heart rate for full minute (both apical and peripheral pulses); note rate, quality, rhythm, pulse deficit
          (2) Assess BP while child is at rest; use properly sized cuff
          (3) Administer cardiac glycosides as ordered; monitor for signs of digoxin toxicity; withhold if pulse falls below or above set limits for the age of the child or if vomiting occurs
          (4) Maintain cardiac monitor
          (5) Position child in semifowler's position to reduce the effort of breathing
          (6) Allow rest periods between activities; provide calm and quiet environment
    2. Acute care: postsurgical
      a. Nursing diagnosis: risk for infection
      b. Expected outcome: prevention of exposure to infection with absence of infection

    c. Interventions
        (1) Use proper hand-washing technique
        (2) Assess child's temperature for elevation, WBC count for an increase, and changes in vital signs (increased HR and RR)
        (3) Monitor condition of incisional and IV sites for signs of infection
        (4) Have child avoid contact with visitors and staff who have infections
        (5) Administer antibiotics as ordered
        (6) Maintain optimum nutrition: encourage well-balanced diet; for infants allow 30 to 45 minutes for feeding; provide a soft nipple to increase fluid intake; monitor daily weight

3. Home care
    a. Nursing diagnosis: altered family processes
    b. Expected outcomes
        (1) Maintenance of support system for family members
        (2) Increased development of coping skills
    c. Interventions
        (1) Assess coping ability and level of anxiety of family members
        (2) Assess need for information and support
        (3) Encourage expression of feelings and concerns
        (4) Assist family to identify effective problem-solving techniques
        (5) Provide information regarding disease process, treatments, long-term care
        (6) Have parents correctly perform a return demonstration for the administration of prescribed medications and verbalization of side effects
        (7) Instruct parents regarding normal growth and development for child's age; actions to facilitate growth
        (8) Assist family to determine appropriate physical activity and limitations for child
        (9) Provide clear instructions about when to call physician: unexplained fever, change in child's behavior

H. Evaluation
1. Questions to ask
    a. Tell me about your plans for the child's care at home regarding: medications, activity, school
    b. How do you deal with your anxiety?

2. Family behaviors to observe
   a. Measures taken to ensure prevention of infection
   b. Statements that indicate effective coping techniques utilized
   c. Statements that indicate positive outlook on child's condition
   d. Growth and development advances are appropriate for age and condition
3. Evaluation of expected outcomes
   a. Heart rate, respiratory rate, and blood pressure maintained within 10% of baseline
   b. Adequate cardiac output is maintained
   c. Parents' anxiety levels are reduced
   d. Parents verbalize pertinent findings for the disease process and the treatment

V. Cyanotic heart defects
A. Definition: abnormalities in which unoxygenated blood mixes with oxygenated blood and enters the systemic circulation; these occur as a result of a right-to-left shunt
B. Cyanotic defects according to hemodynamic classification system
   1. Decreased pulmonary blood flow
      a. Tetralogy of Fallot
      b. Tricuspid atresia
   2. Mixed blood flow
      a. Transposition of great vessels (TGV)
      b. Total anomalous pulmonary venous return or communication
      c. Truncus arteriosus
      d. Hypoplastic heart syndrome
C. Etiology and incidence
   1. Unknown in most cases
   2. Factors associated with cyanotic defects (Table 3-3, p. 107)
   3. Most common cyanotic defect: Tetralogy of Fallot—accounts for 3.8% of congenital defects
D. Pathophysiology
   1. Tetralogy of Fallot (Figure 3-10)
      a. Defect consists of four anomalies
         (1) Ventricular septal defect
         (2) Pulmonic valve stenosis

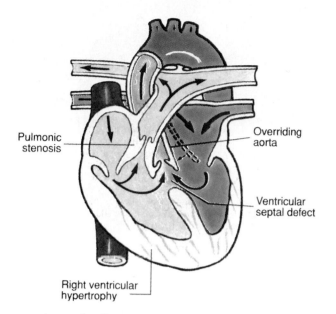

Pulmonic
stenosis

Overriding
aorta

Ventricular
septal defect

Right ventricular
hypertrophy

Figure 3-10. Tetralogy of Fallot. Darker blue areas, saturated blood; darker gray areas, desaturated blood; lighter blue areas, mixed blood. (From Wong, D: *Whaley and Wong's nursing care of infants and children,* ed 5, St Louis, 1995, Mosby.)

        (3) Overriding aorta
        (4) Right ventricular hypertrophy
   b. Defect results in a decreased pulmonary blood flow and right ventricular hypertrophy, with shunting of blood from the right to the left side of the heart
   c. Degree of cyanosis depends on the severity of blood flow obstruction from the right ventricle into the pulmonary artery
  2. Tricuspid atresia
   a. Involves failure of tricuspid valve development, which prevents communication between the right atrium and the right ventricle (Figure 3-11)
   b. Associated with other defects: right ventricular hypoplasia and septal defects
   c. PDA allows pulmonary blood flow for oxygenation; VSD allows a smaller amount of blood to flow to the right ventricle and the pulmonary artery for oxygenation
  3. Transposition of great arteries
   a. Defect involves reversal of two great arteries: the aorta arises from the right ventricle and the pulmonary artery arises from the left ventricle (Figure 3-12)

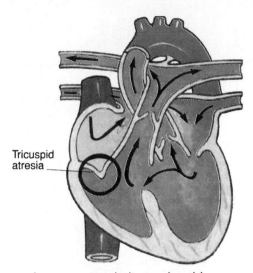

Figure 3-11. Tricuspid atresia (circled). Darker blue areas, saturated blood; darker gray areas, desaturated blood; lighter blue areas, mixed blood. (From Wong, D: *Whaley and Wong's nursing care of infants and children,* ed 5, St Louis, 1995, Mosby.)

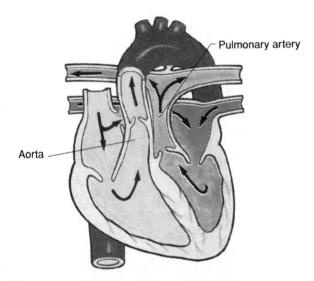

Figure 3-12. Transposition of the great arteries. Blue areas, saturated blood; darker gray areas, desaturated blood. (From Wong, D: *Whaley and Wong's nursing care of infants and children,* ed 5, St Louis, 1995, Mosby.)

    b. Two separate functioning circulatory systems occur: the systemic circulation from the right ventricle and the pulmonary circulation from the left ventricle

    c. Associated defects such as ASD, VSD, and PDA allow mixing of the oxygenated and unoxygenated blood between the two circulatory systems in order to sustain life

    d. Severity of cyanosis is dependent on the amount of blood mixing

4. Total anomalous pulmonary venous return or communication

    a. Defect and failure of the pulmonary veins to join the left atrium; classified according to the pulmonary venous attachment point

        (1) Supracardiac—attachment of the pulmonary veins above the diaphragm (Figure 3-13)

        (2) Cardiac—direct attachment to the heart. Example: right atrium.

        (3) Infracardiac—attachment below the diaphragm. Example: inferior vena cava.

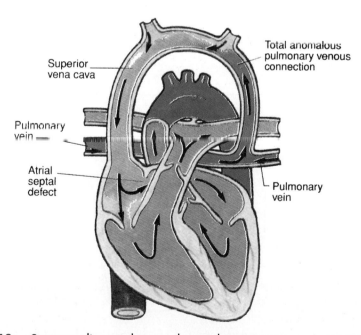

Figure 3-13. Supracardiac total anomalous pulmonary venous connection. (From Wong, D: *Whaley and Wong's nursing care of infants and children*, ed 5, St Louis, 1995, Mosby.)

    b. Since the right atrium receives the majority of blood flow, the right heart hypertrophies

5. Truncus arteriosus
    a. Defect occurs in the embryonic period when the common trunk fails to divide into the pulmonary artery and the aorta; one vessel comes off both ventricles and receives blood from the pulmonary, systemic, and coronary circulations (Figure 3-14)
    b. Three major types of truncus arteriosus
        (1) Type 1: single pulmonary trunk arises from the base of truncus and divides into the left and right pulmonary arteries
        (2) Type 2: right and left pulmonary arteries arise separately from the posterior truncus
        (3) Type 3: pulmonary arteries arise separately from the lateral aspect of the truncus

6. Hypoplastic left heart syndrome
    a. Several complex heart anomalies that involve the left side of heart and include lesions obstructing the systemic blood flow and an underdeveloped aorta, left ventricle, and aortic arch (Figure 3-15)
    b. Results in a return of mixed blood to the right atrium and then shunting from right to left via an ASD

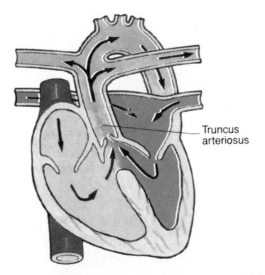

Figure 3-14. Truncus arteriosus. Darker blue areas, saturated blood; darker gray areas, desaturated blood; lighter blue areas, mixed blood. (From Wong, D: *Whaley and Wong's nursing care of infants and children*, ed 5, St Louis, 1995, Mosby.)

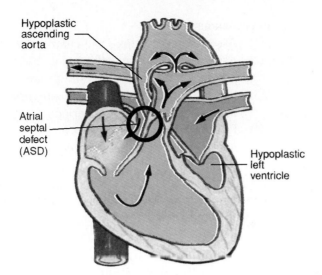

Figure 3-15. Hypoplastic left heart syndrome with ASD (circled). (From Wong, D: *Whaley and Wong's nursing care of infants and children*, ed 5, St Louis, 1995, Mosby.)

E. **Assessment (see Table 3-3, p. 107)**
F. **Therapeutic management**
   1. Medications
      a. Prostaglandins—keep the ductus arteriosus open in premature infants until surgical intervention is possible
      b. Diuretics—promote fluid excretion
      c. Cardiac glycosides—treat CHF
   2. Treatment—conservative until surgery
      c. Surgery (see Table 3-3, p. 107)
G. **Nursing management: child with cyanotic defect**
   1. Acute care
      a. Nursing diagnosis: activity intolerance
      b. Expected outcomes
         (1) Maintain optimal level of activity within limitations imposed by disease process
         (2) Maintain vital signs within predetermined range during activity
         (3) Promote growth and development for age and condition of child

    c. Interventions
       (1) Assess level of fatigue and contributing factors
       (2) Assess vital signs and skin color changes during activity; compare to the resting state
       (3) Provide rest periods between care; prevent disturbances during rest periods
       (4) Provide age-appropriate toys and activities that do not require high energy expenditure
       (5) Provide family with opportunity to share concerns related to activity limitations and care
    d. Nursing diagnosis: risk for injury—complications
    e. Expected outcomes
       (1) Family will identify findings for complications of cardiac defects
       (2) Family will demonstrate technique for safe administration of cardiac medications
    f. Interventions
       (1) Teach family to recognize early signs of drug toxicity and cardiac complications such as right and left heart failure; inform parents when to inform physician
       (2) Teach parents proper administration of cardiac glycoside, times to withhold dose, notify physician
       (3) Have parents perform return demonstrations for proper administration of cardiac glycoside
       (4) Prepare parents for cyanotic episodes; explain rationale for knee-chest or squatting position

2. Home care
    a. Nursing diagnosis: altered growth and development related to limitations in physical activity
    b. Expected outcome: child demonstrates increase in behaviors (personal/social, motor, cognitive) appropriate to age group within limits imposed by disease
    c. Interventions
       (1) Assess child's level of functioning using screening tools such as the Denver II
       (2) Provide stimulation for all the senses: toys and age-appropriate activities within the limits imposed by defect
       (3) Assign consistent caregivers
       (4) Allow the child adequate time to complete tasks and activities for promotion of self-concept and independence

    (5) Provide opportunities to meet age-related developmental tasks

    (6) Teach parents age-related developmental tasks and provide parental guidance information: appropriate setting, provision for discipline, meeting of the child's emotional needs, and selection of age-appropriate activities suited to condition

H. Evaluation

1. Questions to ask
   a. Of what do you need to notify the physician in terms of abnormal findings?
   b. What are your plans for home care: medications, activity level? How will it change when the child goes to day care or school?
2. Behaviors to observe
   a. Child engages in activities appropriate for age and activity level
   b. Parents verbalize the complications to physician
   c. Parents state proper positioning and other interventions for the emergency care of the child to relieve a cyanotic episode
3. Evaluation of expected outcomes
   a. Parents correctly administer prescribed medications and early signs of drug toxicity
   b. Vital signs remain within predetermined limits during activity and at rest

VI. Cardiac surgery

A. Presurgical care

1. Nursing diagnoses
   a. Knowledge deficit
   b. Parental anxiety
2. Expected outcomes
   a. The child and family verbalize knowledge of the basic structure and function of the heart with description of the defect
   b. The child and family state rationale and their role related to various equipment and procedures associated with cardiac surgeries
3. Interventions
   a. Assess the child and the family's readiness to learn
   b. Assess the child and the family's previous experience and present knowledge base

      c. Provide preoperative teaching based on knowledge assessment findings; include visits to the areas where the child and family will be before, during, and after surgery

      d. Use age-appropriate explanations for various procedures and equipment

      e. Encourage the child and family to express feelings and concerns about surgery

      f. Reinforce information provided by the cardiac surgeon or anesthesiologist

B. Postsurgical care

  1. Nursing diagnosis: risk for decreased cardiac output

  2. Expected outcomes: child demonstrates improved cardiovascular function

      a Adequate tissue perfusion

      b. Stabilization of vital signs

      c. Clear lungs upon auscultation

      d. Adequate urine output

  3. Interventions: assess cardiac function

      a. LOC

      b. Vital signs

      c. Central venous pressure

      d. Pulmonary artery pressures

      e. Heart sounds

      f. Peripheral pulses

      g. Renal output

      h. Tissue perfusion

  4. Nursing diagnosis: risk for ineffective airway clearance

  5. Expected outcomes

      a. The child exhibits improved respiratory status

      b. Clear lung sounds and arterial blood gases are within normal limits

  6. Interventions

      a. Monitor rate and depth of respirations, presence of dyspnea and wheezing

      b. Monitor ventilator settings to deliver appropriate tidal volume and oxygen level

      c. Monitor arterial blood gas results

      d. Assess the amount of pulmonary secretions

      e. Monitor chest tube drainage and patency

      f. Turn and suction the child as necessary

      g. Provide chest physiotherapy as ordered

      h. Have the extubated child cough and deep breath q 1 hour

C. **Evaluation**
1. Questions to ask
   a. What are your plans for care of the incision at home?
   b. What are concerns about your child's activity at home?
2. Behaviors to observe
   a. Parents return demonstrate care of incision
   b. Parents facilitate return of child's normal activity level
3. Evaluation of expected outcomes
   a. The child exhibits improved cardiac status including heart rate and blood pressure within normal limits
   b. The child exhibits improved respiratory status including clear lung sounds and arterial blood gases within normal limits for age

VII. Congestive heart failure (CHF)

A. **Description: cardiac disorder in which the heart is unable to deliver adequate blood to the systemic circulation to meet the demands of the body**
B. **Commonly, 90% of infants with congenital cardiac defects develop CHF within first year of life**
C. **Etiology and incidence: CHF is the result of congenital heart disease; other causes for CHF include**
   1. Pulmonary embolism or chronic lung disease
   2. Hemorrhage or anemia
   3. Cardiomyopathies
   4. Severe emotional or physical stress
D. **Pathophysiology**
   1. Basic defect is the decrease in intrinsic contractility of the myocardium, caused by prolonged increased pressure (afterload) or volume overload
   2. Causes classified according to the following changes
      a. Volume overload: left-to-right shunts cause right ventricular hypertrophy
      b. Pressure overload: occurs from obstructive lesions. Example: coarctation of aorta and valvular stenosis.
      c. Decreased contractility: involves disorders that directly affect the contractility of myocardium. Examples: cardiomyopathy and severe anemia.
      d. High cardiac demands: body's need for oxygenated blood exceeds cardiac output. Examples: sepsis, hyperthyroidism.
   3. CHF in children most commonly manifests with bilateral failure; unilateral failure is not typical

4. Compensatory mechanisms are activated as the heart attempts to meet the body's demands
   a. *Cardiac:* hypertrophy and dilatation of the cardiac muscle
   b. *Noncardiac:* sympathetic nervous system stimulation
      (1) Catecholamine release: increased force and rate of myocardial contraction
      (2) Decreased renal perfusion activates renin-angiotensin-aldosterone mechanism to cause retention of water and sodium
5. As compensatory mechanisms fail, CHF findings occur as a result of decreased myocardial contraction and CO, an increased preload and afterload

E. **Assessment**
   1. Assessment findings of CHF can be divided into three groups
      a. Impaired myocardial function
      b. Pulmonary congestion
      c. Systemic venous congestion (Box 3-1, p. 99)
   2. Diagnostic procedures
      a. Laboratory results
         (1) Arterial blood gas values: low PO_2 and pH, high PCO_2
         (2) Serum electrolytes—indicate hyponatremia, hypochloremia, and hyperkalemia
         (3) Digoxin level—monitor for toxicity and regulate dosage; therapeutic level is 0.8 to 2.0 Ng/ml
      b. Diagnostic studies: chest x-ray—reveals cardiomegaly and pulmonary congestion

F. **Therapeutic management**
   1. Medications
      a. Digoxin (Lanoxin)—increase force and decrease rate of cardiac contractions to improve cardiac pumping performance
      b. Diuretics: furosemide (Lasix)—control excessive salt and water retention and decrease preload
      c. Electrolytes: potassium chloride for replacement with diuretic therapy
      d. Sedative/analgesic: morphine to decrease energy expenditure and dilate bronchi
   2. Treatment: medications, light, and diet control
   3. Surgery: unnecessary unless underlying cause needs to be corrected

G. Nursing management
  1. Acute care
    a. Nursing diagnoses
      (1) Decreased cardiac output
      (2) Activity intolerance
    b. Expected outcomes
      (1) Heartbeat is strong, regular, and within limits for age
      (2) Adequate cardiac output, a decrease in the prolonged P-R interval, and a decrease in ventricular rate will be obtained

Age	Range of Heart Rate
1 week to 3 months	100 to 220
3 months to 2 years	80 to 150
2 years to 10 years	70 to 110
10 years to adolescence	55 to 90

      (3) Therapeutic digoxin level (0.8 to 2.0 Ng/ml) will be maintained
      (4) Adequate caloric and protein intake will be provided to support growth
    c. Interventions
      (1) Assess apical heart rate for full minute every 2 hours
      (2) Monitor digoxin level and observe for findings of digoxin toxicity
        (a) Vomiting
        (b) Diarrhea
        (c) Dysrhythmias
      (3) Record strict I&O
      (4) Assess heart sounds and peripheral pulses every 2 hours
      (5) Monitor for potassium levels below 3.5 mEq/L
      (6) Administer diuretics and digoxin as ordered: withhold dose of digoxin if heart rate is <100 beats/min for infant
      (7) Weigh child daily at the same time and in the same clothing, before eating
      (8) Feed infant 2 ounces every 2 to 3 hours as ordered; use gavage feeding if needed
      (9) Allow rest periods after activity
      (10) Add prescribed formula additives such as Polycose, medium-chain triglyceride (MCT) oil as ordered
  2. Home care
    a. Nursing diagnoses

            (1)   Knowledge deficit

            (2)   Anxiety

       b.   Expected outcomes

            (1)   Parents verbalize understanding of infant's condition and treatments

            (2)   Parents demonstrate participation in infant's care including administration of medications

            (3)   Parents verbalize that their anxiety is reduced

       c.   Interventions

            (1)   Assess parents' knowledge level and coping abilities

            (2)   Assess support systems with follow-up referrals

            (3)   Monitor parents' actions with feeding and care; support and make referrals as needed

            (4)   Instruct parents in administration of medications; obtain a return demonstration

            (5)   Instruct parents in CPR or arrange for them to attend formal class

H. Evaluation

   1.   Questions to ask

       a.   What do you need to know about medications and activity at home?

       b.   How have your anxiety and fears decreased?

   2.   Behaviors to observe

       a.   Family's support for and implementation of medical regimen

       b.   Decreased family anxiety as they comply with prescribed follow-up care

   3.   Evaluation of expected outcomes

       a.   Parents verbalize that anxiety regarding child's condition and care are reduced

       b.   Parents verbalize knowledge of the disease process and treatments

       c.   Parents correctly administer the prescribed medications and verbalize initial signs of digoxin toxicity to report to physician

VIII. Acquired heart disease: rheumatic fever

   A.   Description: inflammatory disease following an infection caused by group-A beta hemolytic streptococcus;

   B.   Commonly affects many body systems

       1.   Musculoskeletal: joints—knees, elbows, ankles, wrists

       2.   Cardiac muscle and valves

3. Central nervous system
4. Integumentary

C. Etiology and incidence
1. In majority of cases, an antecedent upper respiratory infection is present 3 weeks before the onset of symptoms
2. May occur at any age; primarily occurs in middle to late childhood
3. Increased frequency among males; seasonal outbreaks observed in late winter and early spring

D. Pathophysiology
1. Streptococci, present in the upper respiratory system, release toxins and enzymes that cause an inflammatory reaction in connective tissue of the heart, joints, and skin
2. Edema and cellular infiltration of the lymphocytes occur
3. Aschoff bodies, rounded nodules containing multinucleated cells and fibroblasts, localize in the mitral valve area of the myocardium

E. Assessment
1. Assessment findings
   a. Polyarthritis—multijoint inflammation
   b. Arthralgia—joint pain
   c. Low-grade fever—99° F to 100° F oral temperature
   d. Chest pain
   e. Chorea—involuntary, purposeless, rapid motions such as raising and lowering the shoulders, grimacing
   f. Macular rash on the trunk and extremities
   g. Subcutaneous nodules in the joints, scalp, and spine
2. Diagnostic procedures
   a. Laboratory results
      (1) Antistreptolysin O titer: elevated
      (2) Erythrocyte sedimentation rate: elevated
      (3) C-reactive protein: elevated
   b. Diagnostic studies
      (1) Diagnosis made by utilizing Jones criteria (Table 3-4, p. 108)
      (2) ECG—identify prolonged PR interval

F. Therapeutic management
1. Medications
   a. Antibiotics—penicillin, erythromycin, benzathine penicillin G, or sulfadiazine as prophylactic therapy against recurrence
   b. Salicylates—decrease inflammation; usually a 2 week course; gradually withdrawn; specifically used in rheumatic

fever; not usually prescribed in the pediatric age group because of the risk of Reye's syndrome

2. Treatments
   a. Bed rest during acute febrile phase
   b. Limit physical exercise in children with carditis
3. Surgery—usually not considered

G. **Nursing management**
1. Acute care
   a. Nursing diagnosis: pain
   b. Expected outcomes
      (1) Joint pain will be relieved or controlled for minimal discomfort
      (2) Child will limit movement that causes discomfort
   c. Interventions
      (1) Assess severity of pain in the joints involved by using pediatric pain scale
      (2) Assess nonverbal signs of pain: crying, irritability, and refusal to move
      (3) Administer analgesics and antiinflammatory agents as ordered
      (4) Maintain bed rest during the acute phase
      (5) Change child's position every 2 hours, maintaining body alignment; move child gently while supporting joints
      (6) Use bed cradle over affected extremities
      (7) Provide age-appropriate quiet activities for diversion
2. Home care
   a. Nursing diagnosis: risk for infection
   b. Expected outcomes
      (1) Child has no reinfection
      (2) Family complies with the medical regimen and follow-up care
      (3) Family notifies the dentist regarding medical history
   c. Interventions
      (1) Instruct parents on the need for prophylactic antibiotic (daily oral, monthly IM) therapy before dental, upper respiratory, and urologic procedures
      (2) Have parents return demonstrate the proper administration of antibiotics
      (3) Assess compliance with the prescribed antibiotic regimen

H. Evaluation
  1. Questions to ask
     a. What is to be done before the application of braces on the child's teeth?
     b. What is your plan for giving medication in school and at home?
  2. Behaviors to observe
     a. Compliance with the antibiotic regimen
     b. Compliance with the methods to protect joints from pain
  3. Evaluation of expected outcomes
     a. Child verbalizes that joint pain is controlled or relieved
     b. Family demonstrates preventive measures to avoid recurrence of disease

Box 3-1. Clinical Manifestations of Congestive Heart Failure

Impaired Myocardial Function

Tachycardia	Anorexia
Sweating (inappropriate)	Pale, cool extremities
Decreased urine output	Weak peripheral pulses
Fatigue	Decreased blood pressure
Weakness	Gallop rhythm
Restlessness	Cardiomegaly

Pulmonary Congestion

Tachypnea	Orthopnea
Dyspnea	Cough, hoarseness
Retractions (infants)	Cyanosis
Flaring nares	Wheezing
Exercise intolerance	Grunting

Systemic Venous Congestion

Weight gain	Ascites
Hepatomegaly	Neck vein distention (children)
Peripheral edema, especially periorbital	

From Wong, D: *Whaley and Wong's nursing care of infants and children,* ed 5, St Louis, 1995, Mosby.

Table 3-1. Commonly used Cardiovascular Medications for Children

Classification	Medication	Indication	Route and Dose		Side Effects	Nursing Implications
Cardiac glycoside, anti-dysrhythmic	Generic: digoxin Trade: Lanoxin	Congestive heart failure Atrial fibrillation	PO *Digitalizing dose* *1-24 months:* 30-50 ug/kg/day in 2 or more doses *2-5 years:* 25-35 ug/kg/day in 2 or more doses *5-10 years:* 15-30 ug/kg/day in 2 or more doses *10 years:* 0.75-1.25 mg in 2 doses	IV 30-50 ug/kg in 3 or more doses 25-35 ug/kg in 3 or more doses 15-30 ug/kg in 3 or more doses 8-12 ug/kg in 3 or more doses	*CNS:* Fatigue, weakness, headache *CV:* Tachycardia, bradycardia, dysrhythmias *GI:* Anorexia, nausea, vomiting *Sensory:* Blurred vision, halos	Monitor VS, ECG Assess serum glycoside level (<2.0 mcg/L) Monitor serum potassium level if also on diuretic Assess hepatic and renal function Administer medications same time daily Take apical pulse for full minute before giving dose Withhold dose if pulse is below normal for age group

			Nursing considerations
Cardiac glycoside, antidysrhythmic —cont'd	PO *Maintenance dose:* *Neonates, infants, and children:* ⅕–⅓ of digitalizing dose daily *10 years and older:* 125-500 ug/kg daily	IV 25%-35% of digitalizing dose in 2-3 daily doses 25%-35% of digitalizing dose once daily	Monitor for signs of digoxin **toxicity:** Tachycardia in young children Bradycardia and upset stomach in older children *Parent teaching:* Teach parent to take pulse for 1 full minute and record before giving medication; hold if HR <110/min or >140/min unless other parameters have been set by physician Teach correct measurement and administration of dose Keep medicine container in locked cabinet Teach signs of CHF

Continued.

Table 3-1. Commonly used Cardiovascular Medications for Children—cont'd

Classification	Medication	Indication	Route and Dose	Side Effects	Nursing Implications
Antidys-rhythmic, calcium channel blocker	Generic: verapamil Trade: Calan, Isoptin	Tachydys-rhythmias Hypertension	PO Not found in pediatric range IV <1 year: 100-200 ug/kg given in 2 min (range 0.75-2 mg) 1-15 years: 100-300 mg/kg given in 2 min (range 2-5 mg)	CNS: Blurred vision, head-ache, weak-ness CV: Tachycardia, hypotension, CHF, bradycardia GI: Nausea, constipation Respiratory: Dyspnea, coughing Hepatic: Hepatotoxicity Integumentary: Rash, hair loss	Monitor for changes from baseline VS Monitor ECG and CVP Infant: CVP 0-4 mm/Hg Child: CVP 2-6 mm/Hg Assess I&O
Antihyper-tensive, B-adrenergic blocker	Generic: propranolol Trade: Inderal	Hypertension (HTN) Supra-ventricular dysrhythmias	PO HTN: 0.5-1 mg/kq/day in 2 doses; increased as necessary to 1-5 mg/ kg/day in 2-4 doses IV 10-20 mg/kg over 10 min	CNS: Insomnia, dizziness, memory changes CV: Bradycardia, hypotension GI: Nausea, vomiting, diarrhea	Monitor CVP, ECG, and BP during IV infusion Nursing actions: Take apical and radial pulse before administering; notify physician of sustained heart rate changes

Antihyper-tensive, B-adrenergic blocker —cont'd			*Respiratory:* Broncho-spasm *Integumentary:* Rash, alopecia	Administer before meals or 2 hours after meals to increase absorption *Parent education:* Teach how to take pulse before administration Weigh child daily and notify physician if increased Give with or between meals
Antihyper-tensive ACE inhibitor	Generic: captopril Trade: Capoten	Hyper-tension Heart failure	PO *Children:* 300 ug/kg tid; increase by 300 ug/kg in 8 to 24 hr intervals prn (children on diuretics or with renal dysfunction should initially receive 150 ug/ kg tid)	*CNS:* Dizziness, headache *CV:* Hypotension, tachycardia, chest pain, palpitations *GI:* Nausea, vomiting, constipation *GU:* Proteinuria, renal dysfunction *Integumentary:* Rash, urticaria	Assess baseline vital signs Take BP before administration Administer 1 hour before meals Take daily weight, I&O Monitor urine for protein *Parent education:* Report weight gain >2 lb/week and edema, especially periorbital

Continued.

Table 3-1. Commonly used Cardiovascular Medications for Children—cont'd

Classification	Medication	Indication	Route and Dose	Side Effects	Nursing Implications
Antihypertensive ACE inhibitor —cont'd				*Hemetology:* Neutropenia, agranulo-cytosis	Monitor serum potassium levels Administer medication 1 hour before meals
Thiazide diuretic	Generic: chloro-thiazide Trade: Diuril	CHF HTN	PO *<2 years:* 125-375 mg/day in divided doses *2-12 years:* 375 mg-1 g/day in divided doses	*CNS:* Headache, dizziness, weakness *CV:* Orthostatic hypotension, weak pulse *GI:* Nausea, vomiting, anorexia, dry mouth *Metabolic:* Hypokalemia, metabolic acidosis *Hematology:* Thrombo-cytopenia *Integumentary:* Rash, photosen-sitivity	Assess baseline VS, especially BP, lying and standing Monitor serum electrolytes, blood glucose, uric acid Assess hydration status, daily weights Monitor for signs of hypokalemia (confusion, weakness, muscle cramps, anorexia) *Parent education:* Administer early in day to prevent nocturia Administer same time daily, encourage potassium-rich foods

Classification	Medication	Use	Dosage	Side Effects	Nursing Considerations
Diuretic, potassium-sparing	Generic: spironolactone Trade: Aldactone	HTN CHF	PO Child 1.5-3.3 mg/kg/day in 1-4 doses	*CNS:* Headache, lethargy, confusion *GI:* Nausea, vomiting, diarrhea *Metabolic:* Hyperkalemia, hyponatremia	Report weight changes to physician: *Infants:* >50 g/24° *Children:* >200 g/24° *Adolescents:* >500 g/24° Child should change position slowly from lying to standing Monitor I&O, daily weights Monitor serum potassium and sodium Monitor BP throughout treatment *Parent education:* Avoid excess intake of potassium in child's diet Teach signs of hyperkalemia (paresthesia, confusion, weakness) Report sore throat, fever, bleeding, or bruising to physician

Table 3-2. Review of Acyanotic Cardiac Defects

Defect	Altered Hemodynamics	Assessment Findings	Therapeutic Management
Ventricular septal defect (VSD)	Oxygenated blood shunted from left to right ventricle	Failure to thrive Frequent respiratory infections	Surgical repair of large VSD Small defects may close with age
Atrial septal defect (ASD)	Oxygenated blood shunted from left to right atrium	Mostly asymptomatic Crescendo-decrescendo, systolic ejection murmur Frequent respiratory infections	Direct surgical closure or suturing in a plastic prosthesis
Patent ductus arteriosus (PDA)	Oxygenated blood shunted from aorta into pulmonary artery	Characteristic machinery-like murmur at middle to left upper sternal border Widened pulse pressure	Surgical repair—surgical division of ligation of patent vessel
Coarctation of aorta	Collateral circulation bypasses coarctated area to supply blood to lower extremities; left ventricular pressure and work load increased	Failure to thrive Weak or absent femoral pulse Systolic murmur Hypertension in upper extremities and lowered BP in lower Fatigue, headaches, leg cramps	Resection of coarcted portion with end-to-end anastomosis of aorta or enlargement of constricted section using graft
Aortic stenosis	Stricture in aortic outflow causes resistance to ejection of blood from left ventricle Elevated left ventricular systolic pressure Left ventricular hypertrophy	Systolic murmur Fatigue, syncope Decreased pulse pressure	Surgical repair—aortic valvotomy

Table 3-3. Review of Cyanotic Cardiac Defects

Defect	Altered Hemodynamics	Assessment Findings	Therapeutic Management
Tetralogy of Fallot	Unsaturated (unoxygenated) blood shunted through VSD directly into aorta Decreased pulmonary blood flow Increased right ventricular pressure	Hypoxemia Cyanosis that increases with activity Hyperkinetic "tet" spells (see triscuspid atresia below) Systolic murmur Digital clubbing Growth retardation	*Surgical repair:* Complex (VSD closure, resection of stenosis, enlargement of right ventricular output tract) Palliative (for those who are unable to have complete repair) involves increasing of pulmonary blood flow (Blalock-Taussig shunting procedure)
Tricuspid atresia	Decreased pulmonary blood flow and increased left-to-right shunting	Cyanosis present at birth Tachypnea, dyspnea, hyperkinetic spells—"blue spells," "tet" spells ▶ Acute cyanosis ▶ Hypernea ▶ Occurs mainly in the morning ▶ May be preceded by crying, feeding Systolic murmur indicative of VSD	Shunt placement to increase blood flow to lungs
Transposition of great arteries	Defect results in two separate circulations Only mixing of saturated (oxygenated) and unsaturated (unoxygenated) blood occurs via defects that may exist ▶ VSD ▶ ASD ▶ PDA	Cyanosis occurs early Hyperkinetic spells CHF	*Surgical repair:* Complete Jotene operation Mustard operation Rastelli procedure Palliative

Table 3-4. Jones' Criteria (Revised) for Guidance in the Diagnosis of Rheumatic Fever

Major Manifestations	Minor Manifestations
Carditis	Clinical
Polyarthritis	Fever
Chorea	Arthralgia
Erythema	History of previous RF or rheumatic heart disease
marginatum	Laboratory
Subcutaneous	Increased erythrocyte sedimentation rate
nodules	C-reactive protein
	Leukocytosis
	Anemia
	Prolonged P-R interval on ECG

Supportive evidence of preceding streptococcal infection:
  Recent scarlet fever
  Positive throat culture for group-A β-hemolytic streptococci
  Increased antistreptolysin-O or other streptococcal antibodies

Presence of two major manifestations or one major and two minor manifestations with supportive evidence of recent streptococcal infection indicates a high probability of rheumatic fever.

REVIEW QUESTIONS

1. A mother has been given instructions regarding the administration of Pediatric Lanoxin (digoxin). The physician has ordered the medication to be administered bid. Which of these statements by the parent indicates an understanding of these instructions?
   a. "I'll give the medication with breakfast and lunch"
   b. "I'll mix the medication with formula"
   c. "I'll give another dose if the baby vomits"
   d. "I'll give the medication before meals, 12 hours apart"

2. An 8-year-old is admitted with a possible diagnosis of rheumatic fever. To help establish the diagnosis of rheumatic fever, the nurse should ask which of these questions?
   a. "Did the child recently travel overseas?"
   b. "Did the child have a recent sore throat?"
   c. "Has the child complained of fatigue?"
   d. "Was the child recently exposed to chicken pox?"

3. A presurgical plan of care has been established for a child before corrective surgery for Tetralogy of Fallot. Which of these nursing diagnoses should receive priority in the child's care during the immediate postsurgical period?
   a. Body-image disturbance
   b. Impaired gas exchange
   c. Knowledge deficit
   d. Altered family processes

4. A nurse reviews the laboratory data on a 6-year-old child admitted with rheumatic fever. Which of the following data is consistent with the child's disease process?
   a. Decreased white blood cell count
   b. Elevated hematocrit
   c. Elevated antibody level
   d. Low erythrocyte sedimentation rate

5. An infant recently admitted to the pediatric unit has been diagnosed with a ventricular septal defect. When doing a physical assessment of this infant, the nurse should expect which of these findings?
   a. Cyanosis, increased anterior-posterior diameter of chest
   b. Extreme difficulty feeding, irritability
   c. Machinelike murmur, shortness of breath
   d. Systolic murmur, no other significant signs

6. A child diagnosed with rheumatic fever is prescribed aspirin. The purpose of this medication is to
   a. Decrease fever
   b. Prevent headache
   c. Promote relaxation
   d. Reduce inflammation

7. A 3-month-old infant is brought to the emergency department. His mother states that he was having trouble feeding and experiencing coughing and irregular breathing. The nurse assesses a respiratory rate of 60 with sternal retractions and an apical rate of 168. An x-ray reveals enlargement of the heart. Which of the following nursing diagnoses should receive priority in this infant's plan of care?
   a. Altered growth and development
   b. Altered nutrition
   c. Decreased cardiac output
   d. Knowledge deficit

8. A toddler has been diagnosed as having coarctation of the aorta. Considering the child's diagnosis, the nurse should expect which of these findings?
   a. Bounding femoral pulses
   b. Blood pressure higher in upper extremities
   c. Machine-like murmur
   d. Weak, thready radial pulse

9. The nurse evaluates the need for further parent teaching regarding long-term antibiotic therapy for a child with rhematic fever based on which of these statements?
   a. "Giving this medication will prevent streptococcal infections."
   b. "Giving this medication will reverse any joint damage that has already occurred."
   c. "We must notify the dentist of this problem before having dental work done."
   d. "We will return to the physician for follow-up injections of penicillin as ordered."

10. Following surgical correction for Tetralogy of Fallot, which of these goals should receive priority in a child's care?
    a. Adequate sleep and rest periods provided
    b. Adequate nutrition
    c. Pain management
    d. Prevention of vascular complications

11. An infant is diagnosed with congestive heart failure. Pediatric Lanoxin (digoxin) is prescribed. The teaching plan for medication administration should include the signs of digoxin toxicity, which are
    a. Apical pulse rate of 90, vomiting
    b. Tachycardia, tachypnea
    c. Fatigue, diaphoresis
    d. Wheezing, pallor

ANSWERS, RATIONALES, AND TEST-TAKING TIPS

Rationales	Test-Taking Tips

1. Correct answer: d

Digoxin administration guidelines include giving the medication at regular intervals, usually 12 hours apart, and 1 hour before or 2 hours after feedings. Digoxin is given on an empty stomach for best absorption, 1 hour before or 2 hours after feedings. Medication is not mixed with the formula, since refusal to take the entire amount results in an inaccurate intake of the dose. If the child vomits, Digoxin guidelines indicate a second dose should not be given.

If you have no idea of the correct response, select the answer that is the most complete, response *d*.

2. Correct answer: b

Research findings support that a relationship exists between upper respiratory infections and group-A streptococci, a frequent cause of sore throats in children, and rheumatic fever (RF). Although RF remains a problem in third-world countries, the etiology is an autoimmune process. Fatigue is a nonspecific finding of many disease processes. Evidence supports a link between the viral disorder, chicken pox and RF. However, RF is caused by bacteria and chicken pox results from a virus.

Approach the question with the association that RF is an inflammation and then select the response that matches with a cause or finding of inflammation, response *b*, sore throat.

3. **Correct answer: b**

Using Maslow's hierarchy to prioritize, physiologic needs take priority over psychosocial needs. The need for gas exchange is the priority physiologic need. Psychosocial needs are not a priority in the immediate postoperative period.

Cluster responses *a, c,* and *d* under psychological needs. Select the remaining response *b,* a physiological need in the immediate postoperative period. The time frame is important to note in this question; it helps further define the correct answer.

4. **Correct answer: c**

Increased Antistreptolysin-O or other streptococcal antibodies are considered reliable indicators of a recent streptococcal infection. An antibody level is also called an antibody titer. In options *a* and *b,* the findings are inconsistent with RF. Erythrocyte sedimentation rate is increased in RF.

Erythrocyte sedimentation rate is also called a sed rate. It is typically elevated when the body has some type of abnormal process—viral or bacterial—occurring.

5. **Correct answer: d**

One of the characteristic signs of ventricular septal defect is a loud, harsh, pansystolic murmur heard best at the lower left sternal border. The findings in option *a* are consistent with cystic fibrosis. The findings in option *b* are consistent with CHF and/or abnormal gastrointestinal conditions. The findings in option *c* are consistent with patent ductus arteriosus (PDA)— the turbulent flow of blood from the aorta through the PDA to the pulmonary artery; this abnormality

The approach to this question is to eliminate the other responses by relating them to conditions; see rationale.

results in a characteristic machinery-like murmur and shortness of breath in a child.

6. Correct answer: d

Salicylates are used to control or minimize inflammation, especially in joints. Although salicylates are effective in decreasing fever associated with the disease process, the primary purpose is to decrease inflammation that can cause pathologic connective tissue changes. Headache is not a major finding associated with rheumatic fever. Aspirin has no relaxation effects.

Recall that a major problem in rheumatic fever is joint inflammation. Associate this effect with rheumatoid arthritis in which ASA is used effectively for controlling the inflammation in the joints. From this effect the relief of pain is a secondary gain.

7. Correct answer: c

The goals for an infant with congestive heart failure (CHF) are to improve cardiac function, remove accumulated fluid and sodium, and decrease the cardiac workload. Achievement of these goals will improve cardiac output. As a result of poor weight gain and activity intolerance, infants with CHF may demonstrate developmental delays; however, it is not a priority in an emergency situation. In addition, there are no data in the stem to support the selection of any of these other nursing diagnoses.

Key words in the stem that indicate an immediate physiological need are "sternal retractions," "respirations of 60," "heart rate of 168," and "enlarged heart." All these data point to an immediate physiological need. The only given physiological response is response c, decreased cardiac output.

8. Correct answer: b

Coarctation of the aorta (COA), a narrowing of the aorta, is usually first identified at a routine physical examination by upper extremity hypertension. In those body areas that receive blood from vessels proximal to the defect, the BP is high and the pulses are bounding. The site of the narrowing is usually the thoracic or the descending aorta. Femoral pulses are weak or absent in coarctation of the aorta. The finding in option *b* is characteristic of patent ductus arteriosus. In COA the pulses are bounding in the body areas that receive blood from vessels proximal to the narrowed aorta.

Eliminate option *c* since the problem is in the aorta and it is unlikely to find a murmur here. Eliminate option *a* by using an educated guess that problems in the aorta will more likely result in weak femoral pulses, not pounding pulses. Eliminate option *d* since it is narrow and only includes the radial pulse. Select option *b*.

9. Correct answer: b

Pathologic changes in joints caused by edema and inflammation are reversible, just as any other inflammation or edema. However, this is not the purpose of long-term antibiotic therapy. The purpose of long-term antibiotics is to prevent further infection. The statements in options *a, c,* and *d* indicate correct knowledge with no need for further teaching. Antibiotic regimens are used to prevent recurrence of RF. Families must be aware of the need

Approach this question by carefully reading the question—which indicates a need for further teaching—and the responses, especially *a* and *b,* "giving this medication;" antibiotic therapy is used with treatment or prevention of infections. Select *b* since reversal of joint damage is done by the body's normal physiologic processes, not by antibiotics.

for continuing antibiotic prophylaxis for dental work and invasive procedures. Prophylactic treatment against recurrence is started after acute therapy and may involve monthly IM injections of penicillin.

10. Correct answer: c

For any postsurgical client, pain management is a priority. Following extubation and removal of tubes, pain can be satisfactorily controlled with PO analgesics. The item in option *a* is an appropriate goal when the concern is to decrease cardiac workload and promote healing. Food and fluids are advanced as with other postoperative clients. The nurse must monitor for signs of hemorrhage, since vascular surgery creates a higher risk for bleeding.

Associate this situation to similar postsurgical clients in which pain management is the initial consideration.

11. Correct answer: a

Principal manifestations of digoxin toxicity in infants are cardiac abnormalities, typically the heart rate—an early sign is bradycardia. The earliest manifestation of "extracardiac" toxicity is vomiting. An infant would not be able to report anorexia. Tachycardia and tachypnea are early signs of CHF, not digoxin toxicity. Fatigue and irritability are signs of CHF. The findings in option *d* are not consistent with digoxin toxicity.

Approach this question by noting that the client is an infant, then make the correct decision.

Nursing Care of Children with Hematological and Immunological Disorders

STUDY OUTCOMES

After completing this chapter the reader will be able to do the following:

▼ Discuss with colleagues the key terms listed.

▼ Describe the major functions of the various blood elements.

▼ Describe the pathophysiology and nursing care of children with sickle cell anemia.

▼ Outline a teaching plan for a child with hemophilia.

▼ Describe the nursing care of children with leukemia and aplastic anemia.

▼ Summarize the pathophysiology and management of acquired immunodeficiency disorder.

KEY TERMS

Anaphylactic hypersensitivity	IgE- or IgG-dependent, immediate-acting humoral hypersensitivity response to an exogenous antigen.
Cell-mediated immunity	Delayed type IV hypersensitivity reaction, mediated primarily by sensitized T cell lymphocytes as opposed to antibodies; responsible for defense against certain bacterial, fungal, and viral pathogens, malignant cells, and other foreign protein or tissue.
Erythrocyte	Also called **red blood cell.** Major cellular element of the circulating blood containing hemoglobin confined within a lipoid membrane; principal function is to transport oxygen; normally lives 110 to 120 days after which it is removed from the blood stream and broken down by the reticuloendothelial system in the liver.
Hemarthrosis	Also called **hemoarthros.** The extravasation of blood into a joint.
Humoral immunity	One of two forms of immunity that responds to antigens; results from the development and the continuing presence of circulating antibodies, produced by the plasma or B cell lymphocytes; antibodies are carried in imunoglobulins IgA, IgG, and IgM.
Leukocyte	White blood cell that functions as a phagocyte of bacteria, fungi, and viruses; five types of leukocytes are classified by the presence or absence of granules in the cytoplasm of the cell— agranulocytes (1) lymphocytes, (2) monocytes and granulocytes, (3) neutrophils, (4) basophils, and (5) eosinophils.
Platelet	Smallest cell in the blood that contains no hemoglobin and is essential for the coagulation of blood and to maintain hemostasis.

CONTENT REVIEW

I. Overview of hematologic system

A. Review of anatomy and physiology

1. The hematologic system includes blood and blood-forming tissue

    a. Two components of blood
- (1) Plasma—the fluid portion, including the solutes
  - (a) Albumin
  - (b) Electrolytes
  - (c) Proteins—clotting factors, globulins, antibodies, fibrinogen
- (2) Formed elements—cellular portion
  - (a) Erythrocytes (RBC)
  - (b) Leukocytes (WBC)
  - (c) Platelets (thrombocytes)

    b. Blood-forming organs
- (1) Red bone marrow or myeloid tissue
- (2) Lymphatic system
  - (a) Lymph
  - (b) Lymphatic vessels
  - (c) Lymphatic structures—thymus, tonsils, spleen, and lymph nodes

    c. All formed elements of the blood are formed in myeloid tissue in postnatal life

    d. Bones of infants and children contain red marrow; following adolescence, only the ribs, sternum, vertebrae, and pelvis produce cells; the remainder of bone marrow becomes yellow from fat deposits

2. Function of the hematologic system and its formed elements

    a. This complex system is responsible for oxygenation of cells, removal of end products of metabolism, immune protection, clotting and heat regulation

    b. Functions of erythrocytes
- (1) Transports hemoglobin, which provides oxygen to cells
- (2) Hemoglobin portion acts as acid-base buffer
- (3) Carbonic anhydrase allows CO_2 to react with blood to be transported to the lungs

    c. Functions of leukocytes
- (1) Neutrophils and monocytes are phagocytes involved in inflammatory reactions
- (2) Eosinophils—involved in allergic or hypersensitivity reactions
- (3) Basophils—responsible for histamine release that increases blood vessel permeability to WBCs at the site of an injury

    d. Functions of platelets
- (1) Clot formation

        (2) Releases serotonin, a vasoconstrictor, at the site of injury to decrease blood flow

B. Assessment

1. Summary of major laboratory and diagnostic studies
   a. Components of a complete blood count (CBC)
      (1) RBC, hemoglobin (Hgb), and hematocrit (HCT): measures the oxygen-carrying capacity of the blood
      (2) WBC: used to diagnose infection; will elevate
      (3) Differential WBCs: used to diagnose bacterial, fungal, and viral infections
      (4) Mean corpuscular volume and mean corpuscular hemoglobin: used to diagnose iron deficiency anemia
      (5) Platelet count: determines severity of bleeding potential
   b. Diagnostic tests
      (1) Bone marrow aspiration: diagnoses leukemia, aplastic anemia, and thrombocytopenia
      (2) Bone marrow biopsy: allows for a more accurate diagnosis of similar items as in bone marrow aspiration
2. Health history
   a. General considerations
      (1) Activity
         (a) Lack of energy
         (b) Tires easily
         (c) Shortness of breath
      (2) Diet and other factors
         (a) Lack of iron in the diet
         (b) Poor growth, appetite
         (c) Tendency to bruise or bleed easily
         (d) Recurrent infections
         (e) Illness in siblings
   b. Family considerations
      (1) History of bleeding tendencies
      (2) Recent infections
      (3) Malignancy
      (4) Anemia
      (5) Maternal HIV
3. Physical examination—findings provide indication of hematologic dysfunction
   a. Lymph: inspect and palpate the lymph nodes for tenderness and enlargement

      b. Skin: pallor, petechiae, cyanosis, ecchymoses, purpura, clubbing of nails

      c. Oral cavity: pallor, bleeding

      d. Neurologic: lethargy, irritability

      e. GI: hepatosplenomegaly

      f. Musculoskeletal: bone pain, joint swelling and pain

II. Mechanisms of immunity

  A. Functions of the immune system

    1. Responds to foreign substances or antigen with

      a. Nonspecific immune defenses—generalized response to any antigen

      b. Specific immune defenses—responds selectively to antigen

    2. Skin is the first line of defense for protection of the body

  B. Components of immune system

    1. Primary lymphoid organs: thymus, bone marrow

    2. Secondary lymphoid organs: lymph nodes, spleen

  C. Mechanisms of immunity

    1. Humoral immunity—specific mechanism involving antibody production and the B-lymphocyte; immune process occurs outside of cells

    2. Cell-mediated immunity—specific mechanism involving immune processes within the cell mediated by T-lymphocyte; T-lymphocytes functions

      a. Viral, fungal, protozoan, and some bacterial protection

      b. Graft rejection

      c. Skin hypersensitivity

      d. Malignant cell surveillance

III. Anemias

  A. Sickle cell anemia (SCA)

    1. Description: severe, chronic anemic disorder

      a. Homozygous form of a group of inherited diseases in which the normal adult hemoglobin (hemoglobin A) is replaced by a variant form (hemoglobin S)

      b. Abnormal hemoglobin results in abnormal shape and increased fragility of erythrocytes

    2. Incidence

      a. One out of twelve Blacks in United States is the carrier for the sickle cell trait

      b. In addition to the Black population, disease may be present in residents of the Arabian peninsula, Greece, Turkey, and India

3. Mode of transmission: autosomal recessive disorder—both parents must be carriers for sickle cell trait; one out of four chance with each pregnancy that the child will have the disease
4. Pathophysiology
   a. In hemoglobin S, the defect is a substitution of valine for glutamine on the beta polypeptide chain of the globin portion
   b. Erythrocytes containing hemoglobin S (HbS) become sickled in shape in situations of decreased oxygen tension and decreased hydration
   c. Sickled RBCs are crescent-shaped, have reduced oxygen-carrying ability and decreased life span
   d. Sickled RBCs are rigid, cause trapping and increased blood viscosity, capillary stasis and thrombosis; eventually tissue ischemia and necrosis result
   e. Sickle cell crises are periods of exacerbation in which symptoms of the disease are most acute
      (1) Three types of sickle cell crises
         (a) Vasoocclusive—painful episodes marked by vessel occlusion, ischemia, and necrosis
         (b) Splenic sequestration—large quantities of blood pooled in liver and spleen
         (c) Aplastic—decreased RBC production, usually resulting from a virus
      (2) Causes of sickle cell crises
         (a) Infection
         (b) Dehydration
         (c) Hypoxia
         (d) Stress
         (e) High altitude
5. Assessment
   a. Assessment findings: tissue ischemia and necrosis that result from increased blood viscosity and RBC destruction; the following sites are affected (Figure 4-1)
      (1) GI tract: spleen and liver
      (2) Kidneys
      (3) Extremities
      (4) CNS—brain
      (5) Lungs
      (6) Eyes

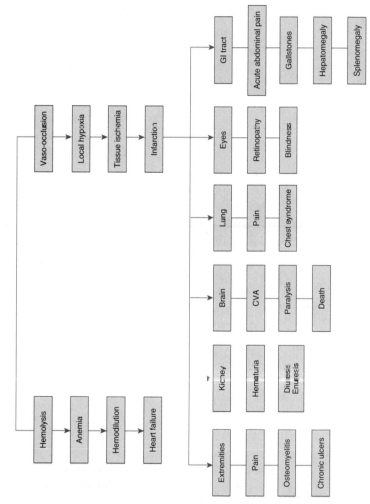

Figure 4-1. Tissue effects of sickle cell anemia. (From Wong, D: *Whaley and Wong's nursing care of infants and children,* ed 5, St Louis, 1995, Mosby.)

    b. Diagnostic procedures: laboratory tests
       (1) Hemoglobin electrophoresis (fingerprinting): detects homozygous and heterozygous forms of the disease and percentages of various hemoglobin forms
       (2) Sickle-turbidity test (sickledex): screening test for hemoglobin S
       (3) Blood smear: may reveal shape of RBC to be sickled rather than normal biconcave disk
       (4) Antenatal screening possible through amniocentesis
    c. Pediatric complications
       (1) Delayed growth, development, and onset of puberty
       (2) Impaired fertility
       (3) Priapism—prolonged or constant penile erection that is painful and infrequently associated with sexual arousal; can result from urinary calculi; caused by microcirculating obstruction and engorgement of the penis; measures to treat: bed rest, sedation— Demerol
       (4) Enuresis—incontinence of urine, especially at night
6. Therapeutic management
    a. Medications
       (1) Analgesics to control the severe pain during crisis
       (2) Antibiotics to treat the existing infection
    b. Treatments
       (1) Rest
       (2) Oxygen administration
       (3) Fluid and electrolyte replacement, usually aggressive
       (4) Blood replacement
    c. Surgery—none
7. Nursing management
    a. Acute care
       (1) Nursing diagnosis: altered tissue perfusion—renal, cerebral, and peripheral
       (2) Expected outcome: optimal circulatory blood flow with delivery of oxygen and nutrients to all organs
       (3) Interventions
          (a) Assess for signs of hypoxia: irritability, restlessness, agitation, hyperventilation, increased apical pulse, and respiratory rates, confusion, cyanosis
          (b) Monitor I&O; priority is to keep well hydrated
          (c) Assess for signs of infection

            (d)   Provide rest periods to decrease oxygen expenditure

            (e)   Administer blood products as ordered; assess for transfusion reaction

       (4)   Nursing diagnosis: pain

       (5)   Expected outcome: child verbalizes absence of or minimal pain

       (6)   Interventions

            (a)   Assess for location, severity, duration, and quality of pain

            (b)   Assess intensity of pain using age-appropriate pain scale

            (c)   Administer analgesics as ordered

            (d)   Apply heat to the affected area

            (e)   Encourage relaxation techniques, deep breathing exercises, and guided imagery

            (f)   Gently handle painful joints and extremities; provide support with pillows

  b. Home care

       (1)   Nursing diagnosis: knowledge deficit

       (2)   Expected outcomes: family possesses knowledge of disease, causes, prevention of crises, and prognosis

       (3)   Interventions

            (a)   Assess knowledge level for SCA: causes, treatments, long-term care

            (b)   Provide age-appropriate explanations to the child and family regarding disease process and treatments

            (c)   Provide emotional support; encourage ventilation of feelings; make referrals to appropriate groups and agencies

            (d)   Provide referral for genetic counseling; encourage screening of family members

8. Evaluation

  a. Questions to ask

       (1)   How does this hospitalization differ from others?

       (2)   What resources do you need at home?

  b. Behaviors to observe

       (1)   Parent's participation in pain evaluation, hydration, and pain-relief measures

       (2)   No evidence of further sickling during assessments

       (3)   Child verbalizes relief of pain

        c. Evaluation of expected outcomes
           (1) Family verbalizes knowledge of disease, cause, and methods to prevent crises
           (2) Family seeks genetic counseling and support from appropriate agencies

B. Aplastic anemia

  1. Description: disorder characterized by bone marrow failure and depletion of all formed elements of blood

  2. Etiology: causes of acquired aplastic anemia
    a. Drugs, including antibiotics and antineoplastic agents
    b. Infection, including hepatitis and human parvovirus
    c. Chemicals: benzenes and petroleum products
    d. Radiation

  3. Incidence
    a. May be acquired or inherited; Fanconi's syndrome is associated with a congenital variety of aplastic anemia
    b. In children, occurs between 3 and 5 years of age

  4. Pathophysiology
    a. Decreased production of blood cells
    b. Replacement of cellular elements of bone marrow with fat
    c. Results in pancytopenia: severe anemia (decreased H&H), leukopenia (decreased WBC), and thrombocytopenia (decreased platelets)

  5. Assessment
    a. Assessment findings
      (1) Petechiae
      (2) Ecchymosis, pallor
      (3) Fatigue
      (4) Recurrent infections
      (5) Bleeding: epistaxis more common
    b. Diagnostic procedures
      (1) Laboratory studies
        (a) CBC—reveals macrocytic anemia
        (b) Platelet—decreased count
      (2) Diagnostic studies: bone marrow aspiration and biopsy; reveals replacement of red bone marrow by fatty, yellow marrow

  6. Therapeutic management
    a. Medications
      (1) Globulins: antilymphocyte (ALG) and antithymocyte (ATG)

        (2) Epoetinalfa (Epogen) therapy: to stimulate erythropoiesis

        (3) Immunosuppressive agents: cytoxan

    b. Treatments

        (1) Total body irradiation

        (2) Transfusion of blood products

    c. Surgery: bone marrow transplantation

  7. Nursing management and evaluation: refer to nursing care of the child with leukemia, pp. 132-133

IV. Hemophilia

A. **Description: a group of blood coagulation disorders that are related to a deficiency of a clotting factor**

  1. Two common forms of hemophilia

    a. Hemophilia A (classic)—deficiency of factor VIII

    b. Hemophilia B (Christmas disease)—deficiency of factor IX

  2. Classified into three groups, according to the severity of factor deficiency: severe, moderate, mild

  3. Hemophilia A accounts for 75% of all cases

B. **Mode of transmission**

  1. Transmitted as X-linked recessive disorder

  2. Frequent pattern of transmission is between an unaffected male and a female who carries the trait for hemophilia

C. **Incidence**

  1. Occurs almost always in males: incidence is 1 in 10,000 male births

  2. Prenatal diagnosis possible through amniocentesis; carrier detection possible

D. **Pathophysiology**

  1. Factors VIII and IX are the plasma proteins necessary for the formation of fibrin clots at the site of vascular injury

  2. The disease is marked by prolonged bleeding into any body tissue

E. **Assessment**

  1. Assessment findings

    a. In infancy

        (1) Prolonged bleeding following circumcision

        (2) Ecchymoses over bony prominences

    b. Throughout life

        (1) Subcutaneous hemorrhages

        (2) Hemarthrosis—bleeding into a joint

             (3) Frequent bruising, bleeding

             (4) Joint pain, stiffness

             (5) Epistaxis

             (6) Bleeding from oral mucosa

      c. Complications

             (1) Airway obstruction as result of bleeding in oral cavity or thorax

             (2) Hepatitis from factor replacement

             (3) Acquired immunodeficiency syndrome (AIDS)

             (4) Muscle atrophy resulting from hemarthrosis

  2. Diagnostic procedures: laboratory studies

      a. Factor assay—reveals deficiency in clotting factors VIII and IX to confirm diagnosis

      b. Coagulation tests: partial thromboplastin time, thrombin clotting time

      c. Coagulation screening: platelet count, bleeding time

      d. Thromboplastin generation test: reveals ability to generate thromboplastin

F. Therapeutic management

  1. Medications

      a. Analgesics/antipyretics to control pain and lower temperature

      b. Nonsteroidal antiinflammatories to decrease inflammation of hemarthrosis

  2. Treatment: factor replacement—administer plasma products such as factor VIII concentrate, cryoprecipitate, and fresh frozen plasma (Table 4-1, p. 138)

G. Nursing management

  1. Acute care/home care

      a. Nursing diagnoses

             (1) Altered protection

             (2) Risk for injury

      b. Expected outcomes

             (1) Prevention of bleeding caused by trauma

             (2) Identification and control of bleeding episodes

      c. Interventions

             (1) Assess for findings of active bleeding, hemarthrosis

             (2) Administer plasma protein, factor replacement, or cryoprecipitate as ordered

             (3) Apply pressure and cold compresses to the site of injury

             (4) Elevate and immobilize affected limb

        (5)   Teach parents symptoms of bleeding: pain, swelling, limited joint motion

        (6)   Teach parents to administer plasma protein when signs of bleeding appear

        (7)   Inform parents of safety precautions: child's wearing of medical identification, providing of a soft toothbrush, avoidance of contact sports, avoidance of aspirin-containing products

        (8)   Encourage selection of iron-rich foods: provide sample menus, food list, dietary consult

   d. Nursing diagnosis: pain

   e. Expected outcome: child verbalizes absence or control of pain

   f. Interventions

        (1)   Assess for joint pain, swelling, and decreased range of motion

        (2)   Administer nonaspirin analgesics, such as acetaminophen, as ordered

        (3)   Immobilize the affected extremity; apply ice to the painful area

        (4)   Use a bed cradle over the affected extremity

   g. Nursing diagnosis: impaired physical mobility

   h. Expected outcomes

        (1)   Child maintains optimal mobility within limitations of the disease

        (2)   Absence of complications of immobility

   i. Interventions

        (1)   Assess mobility status: joint mobility, pain, stiffness, swelling, muscle tone, ability to perform ADLs

        (2)   Assess for appropriateness of activity restrictions and immobility devices (splints)

        (3)   Assess for complications of immobility: skin breakdown, contractures, loss of muscle strength, constipation

        (4)   Provide opportunities for age-appropriate activities, within activity restriction

        (5)   Provide active and passive range of motion exercises q 2 to 4 hours, as needed

        (6)   Inform parents of the need for selected medical and exercise regimens

2. Home care

   a. Nursing diagnosis: altered family processes

   b. Expected outcomes

    (1) Family discusses fears and concerns regarding the genetic disorder

    (2) Staff supports family following diagnosis of hemophilia

  c. Interventions

    (1) Assess the family's coping abilities and any factors influencing this process

    (2) Encourage the family to discuss feelings, anxieties, and guilt related to the transmission of a genetic disorder

    (3) Refer parents for genetic counseling as soon as possible following the diagnosis

    (4) Refer the family to appropriate support groups such as the National Hemophilia Foundation

H. Evaluation

 1. Questions to ask

  a. In preparation for home care, what other information or resources do you need?

  b. What findings do you need to monitor and which ones need to be reported to the physician?

 2. Behaviors to observe

  a. Child verbalizes reduction or absence of pain

  b. Participation in ADLs; absence of complications of immobility

 3. Evaluation of expected outcomes

  a. Parents report signs of bleeding to physician or clinic

  b. Parents state measures to prevent trauma and bleeding episodes

  c. Parents properly adhere to the protocol for administration of concentrates or plasma protein

V. Leukemia

A. Description: term given to a group of malignant diseases of the blood-forming tissue and lymphatics; characterized by the proliferation of immature white cells in the bone marrow

B. Classification

 1. Made according to the prevalent cell type and level of maturity, by use of the following

  a. Lympho—refers to lymphoid or the lymphatic systems

  b. Myelo—refers to involvement of the bone marrow

  c. Blastic and acute—involves immature cells

  d. Cystic and chronic—involves mature cells

2. Two common childhood forms
   a. Acute lymphoid leukemia (ALL)
   b. Acute nonlymphoid or myelogenous leukemia (ANLL or AML)
C. **Etiology and incidence**
   1. Peak onset is between 2 and 6 years of age
   2. ALL is the most common type of childhood cancer; it accounts for one third of the cases of cancer in Caucasian children
D. **Pathophysiology**
   1. Immature WBCs proliferate and invade various organs of the body, particularly the vascular organs, liver, and spleen
   2. Immature cells compete for nutrients with the normal cells and depress the bone marrow function causing
      a. Anemia—from decreased RBCs
      b. Infection—from neutropenia
      c. Bleeding tendencies—from decreased platelets
E. **Assessment**
   1. Assessment findings
      a. From the invasion of bone marrow
         (1) Infection
         (2) Blood in urine and emesis
         (3) Bone weakens and causes fractures; bone pain
         (4) Fever
         (5) Poor wound healing
         (6) Pallor
         (7) Fatigue
         (8) Epistaxis
         (9) Abdominal pain
         (10) Petechiae
      b. From the infiltration of organs
         (1) Hepatosplenomegaly
         (2) CNS: headache, vomiting, increased ICP, lower extremity weakness
   2. Diagnostic procedures
      a. Laboratory tests
         (1) Peripheral blood smear—contains immature WBCs
         (2) CBC—reveals anemia, neutropenia, and thrombocytopenia; done weekly or monthly during maintenance therapy
      b. Diagnostic studies
         (1) Lumbar puncture—assesses CNS involvement
         (2) Bone marrow aspiration—reveals presence of blast cells

          (3)   Bone scan—assesses degree of bone involvement

          (4)   Computerized tomography scan—reveals degree of organ involvement

F. Therapeutic management

   1.   Medications (Table 4-2, pp. 139-140): chemotherapeutic agents—with or without cranial radiation (four levels)

      a.   For induction: to decrease leukemic cells and achieve remission

          (1)   Intravenous vincristine and l-aspariginase

          (2)   Oral prednisone

      b.   For sanctuary: to treat leukemic cells that have invaded the CNS and the testes

          (1)   Intrathecal methotrexate, cytosine, arabinoside, and steroids

          (2)   Irradiation

      c.   For maintenance: follows induction and sanctuary therapy to continue remission

          (1)   Oral 6-mercaptopurine

          (2)   Oral methotrexate

          (3)   Cytarabine

      d.   For reinduction: to reduce the leukemic cells after relapse occurs

          (1)   Prednisone

          (2)   Vincristine

          (3)   Other chemotherapeutic drugs not previously used

      e.   Antigout agents—allopurinol (Zyloprim): to control the severity of hyperuricemia after chemotherapy

   2.   Treatments: radiation, in combination with chemotherapy; as outlined above

   3.   Surgery: bone marrow transplantation

G. Nursing management

   1.   Acute care

      a.   Nursing diagnoses

          (1)   Alteration in nutrition: less than body requirements related to nausea and vomiting associated with chemotherapy

          (2)   Altered oral mucous membrane

      b.   Expected outcomes

          (1)   Side effects of chemotherapy, commonly nausea and vomiting, are minimized or absent

          (2)   Child is protected from exposure to pathogenic organisms

(3) Child's oral mucous membranes remain intact

   c. Interventions

     (1) Use good hand washing technique before and after contact with child

     (2) Assess child for side effects of chemotherapy

     (3) Administer an antiemetic 30 minutes before chemotherapy is ordered; antiemetic commonly continued for up to 1 day after the chemotherapy has been completed

     (4) Assess the oral mucosa for pain, ulcers, lesions, stomatitis, and any effects on eating

     (5) Assess for bleeding from any orifice; check urine and stool for blood; monitor platelet, WBC, Hgb, Hct, and neutrophil count

     (6) Assess for signs of infection

     (7) Provide mouth rinses and soft toothbrush

     (8) Administer topical xylocaine, as ordered, before meals

     (9) Provide bland, soft foods based on child's preference

     (10) Isolate child from individuals with upper respiratory or other infections

     (11) Instruct parents to have child avoid contact sports

     (12) Teach parents to report to physician or clinic any signs of fever, pallor, oozing blood, exposure to a communicable disorder

2. Acute care/home care

   a. Nursing diagnosis: body-image disturbance

   b. Expected outcomes

     (1) Child adapts to limitations of a chronic illness

     (2) Parents seek out social services and psychological counseling as necessary

   c. Interventions

     (1) Assess the family for feelings about a chronic illness with encouragement to express concerns regarding lifestyle changes

     (2) Provide privacy

     (3) Observe the child for signs of withdrawal, regression, or other behavioral changes

     (4) Prepare the family and child for body appearance changes

     (5) Encourage the family to allow the child to participate in safe peer activities

H. Evaluation
1. Questions to ask
   a. What changes will be made in your lifestyle?
   b. How have you prepared for the long-term care?
2. Behaviors to observe
   a. Participation of child in school and peer activities as appropriate
   b. Parents seek out social services or other resources
   c. Compliance by parents and child to prevent breakdown of oral mucosa
3. Evaluation of expected outcomes
   a. Family verbalizes feelings about a chronic disorder with discussion of long-term implications in positive terms
   b. Child's oral mucosa remains intact

VI. Acquired immunodeficiency syndrome (AIDS)

A. **Description: disorder caused by human immunodeficiency virus (HIV) type 1; characterized by a generalized dysfunction of the immune system**
B. **Etiology: the causative agent, HIV, is present in blood and body fluids: semen, saliva, tears, vaginal secretions, and breast milk**
C. Incidence
1. AIDS is the ninth leading cause of death between 1 and 4 years of age; the seventh leading cause of death for adolescents and young adults between 15 and 24 years of age
2. Early cases were identified in sexually active homosexual males; the current risk groups in pediatrics include recipients of multiple transfusions (hemophiliacs) and newborns of affected mothers
D. Pathophysiology
1. HIV infects the helper T lymphocytes, which are responsible for cellular immunity, and lies dormant or proliferates; HIV then inactivates the immunity of that cell
2. In pediatric AIDS, abnormal B cell function is present early in the course of the disease; thus, both the cellular and the humoral immunity are compromised
3. HIV attacks the macrophage and uses the cell to cross the blood-brain barrier
4. Mode of transmission occurs primarily by blood contact or sexual contact

E. **Assessment**
1. Assessment findings
   a. Infants: perinatally affected
      (1) Lymphadenopathy
      (2) Hepatosplenomegaly
      (3) Opportunistic infections
      (4) Progressive encephalopathy
      (5) Microcephaly
   b. Infants: infected during the neonatal period
      (1) Failure to thrive
      (2) Developmental delays
      (3) Oral candidiasis
      (4) Diarrhea
      (5) Hepatosplenomegaly
      (6) Chronic interstitial pneumonia and cough
      (7) Chronic otitis media
   c. Children/adolescents
      (1) Malaise
      (2) Fatigue
      (3) Night sweats
      (4) Weight loss
      (5) Diarrhea
      (6) Fever
      (7) Regression of developmental milestones
      (8) Generalized lymphadenopathy
      (9) Nephropathy
      (10) Interstitial pneumonitis and pneumocystis carinii pneumonia
      (11) Encephalopathy
2. Diagnostic procedures: laboratory studies
   a. Enzyme-linked immunosorbent assay (ELISA)—determines response of antibodies to the HIV virus
   b. Western blot—confirms the presence of HIV antibodies
   c. CBC—reveals increased WBC with infection; decreased helper T cells

F. **Therapeutic management**
1. Medications
   a. Antivirals—acyclovir (Zovirax) to reverse viral replication
   b. Antibiotics—trimethoprim/sulfamethoxalone (Bactrim/Septra) combination to treat opportunist infections
   c. Gamma globulin—to compensate for deficiency of B-lymphocytes

      2. Immunizations: inactivated poliovirus (IPV) is substituted for oral poliovirus (OPV) in the regular immunization schedule

F. Nursing management

  1. Acute care

    a. Nursing diagnosis: risk for infection

    b. Expected outcomes

      (1) Child's risk of future infections is reduced

      (2) Family verbalizes risk factors in acquiring or transmitting the disease

    c. Interventions

      (1) Provide private room; child should avoid exposure to other illnesses

      (2) Wash hands before entering and after leaving room

      (3) Assess for: fever, malaise, fatigue, weight loss, vomiting and diarrhea, altered activity level, oral lesions

      (4) Wear gloves for care; especially when in contact with body fluids and changing diapers

      (5) Label contaminated articles and dispose of them according to the hospital policy and Centers for Disease Control guidelines

      (6) Administer medication—zidovudine (AZT) to minimize disease progression

      (7) Administer gamma globulin monthly to compensate for B-lymphocyte deficiency

    d. Nursing diagnosis: altered nutrition—less than body requirements

    e. Expected outcome: child regains optimal nutritional status

    f. Interventions

      (1) Document child's weight with comparison to previous weight

      (2) Assess oral cavity for presence of candida

      (3) Assess dietary and fluid intake and output

      (4) Monitor serum/urine electrolytes, albumin, glucose

      (5) Provide high-calorie, high-protein diet

      (6) Administer dietary supplements/total parenteral nutrition as ordered

      (7) Administer medications to treat monilial infection

  2. Home care

    a. Nursing diagnosis: social isolation

    b. Expected outcomes

      (1) Child's and family's feelings of isolation are reduced

      (2) Child participates in family and school activities as much as possible

    c. Interventions

        (1) Assess the child and family for feelings of rejection

        (2) Provide an opportunity for the family to express feelings regarding the social stigma of the disease

        (3) Encourage the child to interact with peers; attend school and social activities

        (4) Provide peers and school personnel with information regarding mode of transmission and safe activities for the child

        (5) Be available to answer any questions and concerns

H. Evaluation

  1. Questions to ask

    a. What are your plans for school, social, and home activities?

    b. What are your concerns about long-term needs and medications?

  2. Behaviors to observe

    a. Child participates in family and peer activities

    b. Child attends school within limitations of the disease and treatment

  3. Evaluation of expected outcomes

    a. Child remains free of opportunistic infection

    b. Family and the child exhibit a reduction in anxiety and feelings of isolation

    c. Family seeks assistance from support group

Table 4-1. List of Plasma Products Commonly Used to Treat Children with Hemophilia

Plasma Product	Description of Contents	Indications	Comments
Cryoprecipitated antihemolytic factor (AHC)	All coagulation factors	Hemophilia A Von Willdebrand's disease	Lowers risk of infection
Fresh frozen plasma (FFP)	Factor VIII fibrinogen Contains all plasma-clotting factors	Unknown type of hemophilia Mild hemophilia A or B	Lowers risk of infection IV piggybacked with normal saline
Factor VIII (AHF) concentrate	Factor VIII	Hemophilia A	Higher risk of infection
Factor IX concentrate	Factor IX Factors II, VII, X	Hemophilia B	Higher risk of infection

Modified from Betz and Poster: *Mosby's pediatric nursing reference*, St Louis, 1992, Mosby.

Table 4-2. Summary of Commonly Used Chemotherapeutic Agents in Pediatrics

Agent	Indications	Side Effects	Nursing Implicctions	Route
Actinomycin-D	Wilm's tumor Ewing's sarcoma	Nausea, vomiting, diarrhea Stomatitis Alopecia Thrombocytopenia	Monitor IV infusion to avoid extravasation Monitor vital signs and assess for signs of infection Assess oral mucosa and hemetest stools	IV
Cytosine arabinoside	ALL ANLL Prophylaxis CNS therapy	Nausea, vomiting, anorexia Stomatitis Rash, alopecia Hyperuricemia Hepatotoxicity	Monitor for drug toxicity and infection Monitor liver and kidney function tests—ALT, AST/ creatinine Observe for fluid and electrolyte imbalance	IV, IM, IT (Intrathecal: given into the spinal canal)
DTIC dacarbazine	Neuroblastoma Ewing's sarcoma	Nausea, vomiting Myelosuppression Fatigue, malaise	Monitor infusion to avoid extravasation Administer IV fluids to avoid imbalances Monitor vital signs and observe for infection	IV
L-Asparignase	ALL induction	Nausea, vomiting Headache, fever Anaphylaxis Liver function impairment	Observe for 30-60 minutes upon initiating medication for signs of anaphylaxis Monitor liver function test Increase fluid intake	IM, IV

Continued.

139

Table 4-2. **Summary of Commonly Used Chemotherapeutic Agents in Pediatrics—cont'd**

Agent	Indications	Side Effects	Nursing Implications	Route
6 MP mercapto-purine	ALL maintenance therapy	Leukopenia GI ulceration Jaundice Rash, pigmentation	Assess baseline liver function Observe for signs of infection Recommend good oral hygiene Observe for signs of bleeding	PO
Methotrexate	ALL	Photosensitivity Myelosuppression Hepatotoxicity (at high-dose therapy)	Assess baseline hepatic function Avoid vitamins, tetracycline, Dilantin, chloramphenicol Avoid exposure to ultraviolet light	PO, IV, IM, IT (Intrathecal: given into the spinal canal)
Prednisone	ALL maintenance therapy	Weight gain Cushing's states Hypertension Impaired wound healing	Obtain baseline height and weight Report any sudden weight gain Teach family not to stop drug abruptly Encourage diet low in sodium	PO
Vincristine	ALL maintenance therapy Neuroblastoma	Neurotoxicity Constipation Leukopenia Liver toxicity Paralytic ileus	Assess baseline CBC and bilirubin Monitor I&O, weight Assess neurologic status Assess vital signs Assess bowel elimination	IV
Adriamycin	Wilm's tumor Neuroblastoma	Nausea, vomiting Stomatitis Alopecia ECG changes	Assess baseline ECG Monitor IV site for extravasation Instruct patient that urine may turn red for 48 hours after infusion	IV

REVIEW QUESTIONS

1. A 12-year-old hemophiliac client has been admitted to the medical center for an acute episode of hemarthrosis. Which of these expected outcomes should receive priority in the client's care?
   a. Family will receive genetic counseling
   b. Maximum function of the joint will be restored
   c. Child and family will seek support from National Hemophilia Foundation
   d. Child will participate in appropriate activities for present condition

2. A child with leukemia complains of fatigue. The nurse assesses the skin color as pallor. Considering the child's diagnosis, which of the following data explain these findings?
   a. Cerebrospinal fluid with elevated white cells
   b. Hemoglobin of 8 g/dl
   c. Platelet count of 150,000/mm^3
   d. Sodium level of 130

3. A 9-year-old with sickle cell anemia has been hospitalized in vasoocclusive crisis. Because the child complains of painful joints, which of these actions should the nurse take to promote the child's comfort?
   a. Apply ice compresses and elevate the affected extremities
   b. Apply heat packs and administer an ordered analgesic
   c. Provide cold compresses and administer aspirin
   d. Provide heat packs and passive range of motion

4. A hemophiliac has been diagnosed with acquired immunodeficiency syndrome (AIDS). In response to the parents' questions about the probable mode of transmission, which of these statements is most correct about the mode of transmission in their child?
   a. Contact with a child with varicella virus
   b. Contaminated factor VIII replacement
   c. Recent immunization
   d. Casual contact with child known to have HIV

5. To promote optimal functioning of a 14-year-old child with hemoarthrosis, the nurse's best action would be to
   a. Elevate and immobilize the affected joint
   b. Institute passive range of motion to the affected joint during acute phase
   c. Apply pressure to the area as needed
   d. Apply warm compresses to the affected joint

6. Which of the following nursing diagnoses should receive priority during a vasoocclusive crisis in a 14-year-old with sickle cell anemia?
   a. Decreased cardiac output
   b. Ineffective individual coping
   c. Alteration in comfort
   d. Ineffective airway clearance

7. Which of these instructions should the parents of a child who has recovered from a sickle cell crisis receive?
   a. Avoid contact with all children
   b. Isolate child from known sources of infection
   c. Restrict child's intake during the night
   d. Reinforce the basics of trait transmission

8. Methotrexate was administered into the spinal canal of a 6-year-old diagnosed with leukemia. The nurse explains to the parents that this drug was given
   a. Intraosseous
   b. Intrathecal
   c. Dermal
   d. Lingual

9. Which of the following nursing diagnoses should be part of a hemophiliac's long-term plan of care?
   a. Altered health maintenance
   b. Risk for injury
   c. Social isolation
   d. Anticipatory grieving

10. Methotrexate is classified as an antimetabolite. When teaching the parents about how this medication works, the nurse includes the following information
    a. It lowers uric acid concentration, which occurs after chemotherapy and radiation
    b. It interferes with folic acid metabolism, which is essential for synthesis of nucleoproteins required by rapidly dividing cells
    c. It suppresses the bone marrow that produces the formed elements of the blood
    d. It decreases the level of amino acid necessary for tumor growth

ANSWERS, RATIONALES, AND TEST-TAKING TIPS

Rationales   **Test-Taking Tips**

1. Correct answer: b

Repeated hemarthroses may result in incomplete absorption of the blood in the joints. Flexion contractures and joint fixation may occur from limitations of range and motion, as well as bone and muscle changes. Options *a,* *c,* and *d* are incorrect as priorities. Psychosocial needs are appropriate to the care plan; however, restoration of physical conditions take top priority.

Approach this question by using Maslow's hierarchy of needs, with physiological needs being met first.

2. Correct answer: b

In leukemia, bone marrow is infiltrated with proliferative immature cells. Decreased red blood cell production results in decreased hemoglobin and a diagnosis of anemia. The finding in option *a* is consistent with meningitis. The platelet count is within normal range, beginning at 150,000/mm³. A decreased platelet count, thrombocytopenia, has findings of bleeding or hemorrhage. A high count, thrombocytosis, has findings of clot formation such as thrombophlebitis of the legs. A decrease in the serum

Remember that clinical findings of skin pallor, fatigue, and shortness of breath are classic complaints of clients with anemia.

sodium does not result in pallor or fatigue. Clinical findings of low serum sodium include confusion, hostility, and agitation.

3. Correct answer: b

Pain management includes analgesics, initial acetaminophen, and the application of heat. Cold or ice compresses are not applied to the area because the cold enhances sickling of the red cells and local vasoconstriction. Passive range of motion promotes circulation; however, the child's activity tolerance will dictate whether passive exercises are possible. Information given in the stem indicates the child is presently in pain, at which time any exercises would be contraindicated.

Heat dilates and improves circulation, especially when the cells are sickled. As with any client in pain, provision of medication for maximum relief of pain is a priority.

4. Correct answer: b

In the pediatric population, children who have received blood products, especially children with hemophilia who have received multiple blood products, are at risk. HIV is transmitted through direct contact with blood or blood products. Neither varicella virus, which causes chicken pox, nor recent immunization cause AIDS. There is no evidence that casual contact between

Approach this question by eliminating the responses you know are incorrect; then select the remaining one.

affected and unaffected individuals can spread the HIV virus.

5. **Correct answer: a**

During bleeding episodes, the joint is elevated and immobilized to prevent crippling effects of joint degeneration, which is a specific problem with hemarthrosis. Passive range of motion exercises start after the acute phase. The response in option *c* is too general to be correct. Pressure to the area must be applied for at least 10 to 15 minutes to allow for clot formation. Cold instead of warm packs or compresses are used to promote vasoconstriction to stop or minimize the bleeding.

Apply basic principles for care of a damaged extremity—elevate and immobilize.

6. **Correct answer: c**

Vasoocclusive crises are the result of sickled cells obstructing the blood vessels, causing an occlusion with the results of ischemia and necrosis. The affected extremities are most painful during this acute sickle cell crisis. Comfort is a priority. The nursing diagnoses in options *a* and *d* are inappropriate to use with the condition of a vasoocclusive crisis. There is insufficient data in option *b* to support this as a nursing diagnosis.

Key words in the stem are "vaso-occlusive crisis;" associate this crisis with other conditions in which there is occlusion of the vessel such as angina. This leads to the selection of response *c*, which is also a priority for the client with angina.

7. **Correct answer: b**

Infection is the major predisposing factor in the development of sickle cell crisis. During the infection and stress of the sickle cell crisis, the body's immune system is compromised. The parents should understand the need to isolate the child from known sources of infection for at least a few weeks after hospitalization, until the immune system is recovered. Parents must understand the need to balance the developmental needs of the child and to model living a normal life. Hydration is necessary for hemodilution, which prevents sickling. Fluids are not restricted. The action in option *d* is an appropriate intervention following the initial diagnosis when the child is old enough to understand the process.

Eliminate response *a,* since it has the absolute "all" in it; this would be impossible to achieve. Eliminate response *c,* since there are only a few situations in which fluids are restricted—increased intracranial pressure, renal failure, and wetting the bed at night. Responses *d* and *b* sound like good choices. One way to select the correct answer is reread the stem. Note that an age is not given; therefore, response *d* is probably incorrect, since an age would clue one into the ability of the child to understand. A second method is to select response *b,* since the physiological need has priority over the psychosocial need.

8. **Correct answer: b**

Intrathecal Methotrexate is directed to act in the central nervous system and is protected by the blood-brain barrier. Intraosseous route provides an alternate route for the administration of fluids and medications until intravascular access can be attained. A needle is inserted into the medullary cavity of the long bone, most often the distal femur or proximal

Use association to make your selection: lingual with tongue, dermal with skin, and osseous with ossification or bone. Thus, the only response left is *b.*

tibia. Medication is administered between the skin layers below the surface stratum corneum. Tablets dissolve in the mouth—lingual under the tongue; medication is absorbed directly into the blood stream.

9. Correct answer: b

With hemophilia, hemorrhage can occur as a result of minor trauma such as a slight fall or bruise. Ultimate prognosis for the child depends on the family's ability to learn effective methods of prevention of physical injury and to balance child rearing practices with injury protection.

Apply Maslow's hierarchy of needs: physical needs supersede psychosocial needs. Therefore, response *b* is the only diagnosis for physical needs and is the best selection.

10. Correct answer: b

Methotrexate inhibits the action of dehydrofolate reductose, thereby blocking normal biochemical reactions and inhibiting DNA and RNA synthesis of rapidly acting cells. Option *a* describes the action of allopurinol (Zyloprim), which is useful in preventing hyperuricemia in clients who are receiving cancer chemotherapy. Option *c* describes the side effect of various chemotherapy drugs and radiation therapies for cancer. Option *d* describes the action and indication for the pyrimidine analogues.

Associate methotrexate with antineoplastic drugs. Then reread the responses and narrow the answer to either *b,* which has the words "rapidly dividing cells," and *d,* which has the words "tumor growth." Select response *b,* which is more specific in the description of cancer cells.

Nursing Care of Children with Respiratory Disorders

STUDY OUTCOMES

After completing this chapter, the reader will be able to do
the following:

▼ Discuss with colleagues the key terms listed.

▼ Compare acute otitis media and otitis media with effusion with
regard to pathophysiology, clinical manifestations, therapeutic
management, and nursing management.

▼ Differentiate among the major types of upper and lower airway
infections.

▼ Compare various types of pneumonia.

▼ Outline a teaching plan for home care management of a child with
cystic fibrosis.

▼ State rationale for various treatment modalities indicated for a child
with acute asthma.

KEY TERMS

Arterial oxygen tension (PaO_2)	Force with which oxygen molecules, physically dissolved in blood, are constantly trying to escape, expressed as partial pressure, PaO_2; normal = 80 to 100; for COPD clients = 60 to 80.
Humidification	Process of increasing the relative humidity of the atmosphere around a client through the use of aerosol generators or steam inhalers that exert an antitussive, cough inhibitor effect; acts by decreasing the viscosity of bronchial secretions.
Influenza	Highly contagious infection of the respiratory tract caused by a myxovirus and transmitted by airborne droplet infection; incubation period 1 to 3 days followed by sudden onset of fever, chills, and malaise; complete recovery in 3 to 10 days after symptomatic treatment; fever and constitutional symptoms distinguish it from the common cold.
Partial pressure of CO_2 ($PaCO_2$)	Portion of total blood gas pressure exerted by carbon dioxide; normal = 35 to 45.
Status asthmaticus	Acute, severe, and prolonged asthma attack.
Stridor	Abnormal, high-pitched, musical sound caused by an obstruction of the trachea or larynx; usually heard during inspiration.
Upper respiratory infection (URI)	Infection located from the trachea upward in the respiratory tract; usually includes the common cold, laryngitis, pharyngitis, rhinitis, sinusitis, and tonsillitis.
Wheeze	Sound characterized by a high-pitched musical quality; caused by a high-velocity flow of air through narrowed bronchi; may be heard both during inspiration and expiration.

CONTENT REVIEW

I. Respiratory system overview

A. Structure

1. Respiratory system is comprised of the following

a. Upper respiratory tract

(1) Nose—serves to filter and moisten air

(2) Pharynx—contains tonsils; responsible for phonation

        b. Considered either upper or lower respiratory tract
            (1) Larynx—cartilaginous framework containing glottis and epiglottis
            (2) Trachea—smooth muscle structure supported by rings of cartilage; divides into two primary bronchi
        c. Lower respiratory tract (the reactive portion)
            (1) Bronchial tree—divides into secondary bronchi as they enter lung; further divide into bronchioles
            (2) Lungs—mainly consists of alveoli; right lung has three lobes; left lung has two lobes

2. Alveoli, the sites of gas exchange, are located within the lobules of the lungs; the space up to the alveoli is called dead space—meaning no gas exchange takes place
3. Pulmonary capillaries surround the alveoli
4. The medulla oblongata maintains neurocontrol of breathing
5. The bronchial and pulmonary arteries supply blood to the lungs
6. The phrenic nerve innervates the diaphragm, the major muscle of respiration

B. Functions
1. Primary functions of respiratory structures are to supply oxygen to the cells and remove carbon dioxide, the end product of metabolism
2. The upper respiratory tract (URT) allows air into the lower respiratory tract; URT purifies and humidifies the air
3. Mechanism of gas exchange occurs across alveolar membrane to pulmonary capillaries
4. The lungs serve as a buffering mechanism for altering CO_2 to maintain acid-base balance
5. Gas exchange occurs as result of three processes
    a. Ventilation—inhalation and expiration
    b. Diffusion—movement of gases across alveolar membrane dependent on pressure gradient from areas of high to low concentration
    c. Perfusion—oxygenated blood is transported from lungs to tissues of the body

C. Pediatric considerations
1. Major anatomical differences that affect the way infants and children respond to respiratory pathology
    a. Peripheral airways narrowly branch, causing easier airway obstruction
    b. Less alveolar area is available for gas exchange

      c. Eustachian tube is in a more horizontal plane; tubes are shorter, wider, and straighter; this increases risk of infection, peak between 6 months and 2 years of age

      d. Right bronchi is straighter

D. Assessment

  1. Health history

     a. Focus for general questions

       (1) Home environment

         (a) Possible allergens

         (b) Exposure to environmental hazards, chemicals, dust, animals, smoke

       (2) Activity

         (a) Exposure to respiratory infections

         (b) Travel to a foreign country

       (3) Medications: current medications for breathing difficulties, allergy problems, ear infections

     b. Present health questions regarding the presence of the following findings

       (1) Coughing

       (2) Shortness of breath

       (3) Tightness in chest

       (4) Nasal congestion, noisy respirations, nasal flaring

       (5) Sudden onset of difficulty breathing, grunting with respirations

       (6) Difficulty feeding

       (7) Apnea

     c. Medical history

       (1) Low birth weight; prematurity; use of ventilation-assistance devices

       (2) Thoracic surgery

       (3) Previous hospitalizations for pulmonary disease

       (4) Hyperactive airway disease

       (5) Chronic pulmonary disorders: cystic fibrosis, tuberculosis

     d. Family history

       (1) Tuberculosis

       (2) Cystic fibrosis

       (3) Allergy, atopic dermatitis

       (4) Smoking

  2. Physical examination

     a. Examination of anterior and posterior chest

       (1) Skin color, chest wall configuration

        (2) Breathing pattern and effort

        (3) Respiratory rate and depth

        (4) Chest movement with breathing—use of accessory muscles, retractions

    b. Palpate chest for

        (1) Thoracic expansion

        (2) Tactile fremitus

        (3) Crepitus, grating sensation

    c. Auscultate chest

        (1) Quality of breath sounds

        (2) Abnormal breath sounds

        (3) Vocal resonance

    d. Nasal passage

        (1) Drainage

        (2) Nasal flaring

  3. Diagnostic procedures

    a. Laboratory studies

        (1) CBC

        (2) Arterial blood gases

        (3) Sputum culture, sputum for acid-fast bacilli

        (4) Throat culture and sensitivity

    b. Diagnostic studies

        (1) Pulmonary function study

        (2) Chest x-ray

        (3) Oximetry

        (4) Bronchoscopy

D. Medications (Table 5-1, pp. 174-177)

II. Infections and croup syndromes of the upper respiratory tract

A. Otitis media

  1. Description: middle ear infection caused by bacteria or virus; a very common disorder of early childhood

  2. Classified as acute otitis media (AOM) or otitis media with effusion (OME)

  3. Etiology

    a. Half of all children experience otitis media by 1 year of age

    b. Causative organisms of AOM: streptococcus pneumonia and hemophilus influenza

    c. Peak incidence occurs between 6 months and 2 years of age

4. Pathophysiology
   a. Malfunction or obstruction of the eustachian tube causes the collection of fluid in the middle ear, negative middle ear pressure, and results in an effusion
   b. Factors that predispose young children to development of otitis media
      (1) Anatomic position of the eustachian tube: shorter, wider, and straighter
      (2) Undeveloped cartilage lining
      (3) Immature humoral defense system
      (4) Feeding position encourages pooling of fluids and formula in pharyngeal cavity
   c. Complications of otitis media
      (1) Chronic otitis media
      (2) Hearing loss
      (3) Meningitis
      (4) Eardrum perforation and scarring
      (5) Cholesteatoma—cystic mass in middle ear
5. Assessment
   a. Assessment findings
      (1) Acute otitis media (AOM)
         (a) Fever, usually around 104° F rectal
         (b) Bulging and bright red tympanic membrane
         (c) Severe pain; smaller children pull at the affected ear
      (2) Otitis media with effusion (OME)
         (a) Fullness in the ear
         (b) Dull and retracted tympanic membrane
         (c) Serous fluid in the middle ear
   b. Diagnostic procedures
      (1) Laboratory studies: culture and sensitivity (C&S) of the purulent discharge for identification of the causative organism
      (2) Diagnostic studies
         (a) Tympanogram—measures the stiffness and the compliance of the tympanic membrane
         (b) Audiometry—assesses the severity of a hearing loss
6. Therapeutic management
   a. AOM
      (1) Medications
         (a) Antibiotics—10 to 14 day regimen to eradicate the causative organism

          (b)   Analgesics/antipyretics—to decrease fever and pain

          (c)   Decongestants—to decrease nasal congestion

      (2)   Treatment: screening for hearing loss; after effective therapy decrease factors for increased risk of infections

      (3)   Surgery: myringotomy—to relieve symptoms

   b.   Home care

      (1)   Medications: antihistamines—decrease drainage and inflammation in the middle ear; clear the eustachian tube

      (2)   Surgery

          (a)   Myringotomy with needle aspiration

          (b)   Insertion of tympanoplasty tubes to facilitate drainage and help ventilate the middle ear

          (c)   Adenoidectomy and/or tonsillectomy, usually if frequent repeated infections

7.   Nursing management

   a.   Acute care

      (1)   Nursing diagnosis: alteration in comfort

      (2)   Expected outcomes

          (a)   Absent or decreased pain after therapy

          (b)   Child's rest needs are met

      (3)   Interventions

          (a)   Assess verbal and nonverbal signs of pain: irritability, tugging at ear, bulging tympanic membrane

          (b)   Administer analgesics as ordered

          (c)   Position for comfort and drainage: lying on affected side

          (d)   Local application of heat

          (e)   Cleanse external canal with sterile swab soaked in hydrogen peroxide

          (f)   Have child avoid chewing during acute period by offering soft diet; chewing increases pain

   b.   Home care

      (1)   Nursing diagnosis: knowledge deficit

      (2)   Expected outcomes

          (a)   Parents verbalize understanding of follow-up care and prevention techniques

          (b)   Child recovers from infection and surgery without complications

        (3) Interventions
           (a) Emphasize need for following prescribed antibiotic regimen
           (b) Teach parents to feed infants in upright position and encourage the older child to play blowing games and chew gum
           (c) Instruct parents to maintain patency of tympanoplasty tubes: keep ears dry—earplugs should be worn during bathing, shampooing, and swimming; diving or submerging under water is not allowed
           (d) Teach parents to observe for signs of hearing impairment

8. Evaluation
   a. Questions to ask
      (1) What is allowed in water activities?
      (2) What are the concerns about the medications needed?
   b. Behaviors to observe
      (1) Child resumes normal activity level
      (2) Parents ask appropriate questions for follow-up care
   c. Evaluation of expected outcomes
      (1) Reinfection of middle ear is prevented
      (2) Child recovers from surgery or infection without complications

B. Epiglottitis
1. Description: acute inflammation of epiglottis involving the supraglottic obstruction; since the condition results in respiratory distress, it is an emergency situation
2. Etiology: caused by a bacterial organism, usually hemophilus influenza; rarely, streptococci
3. Incidence
   a. Most commonly affects children between 3 and 7 years of age
   b. Occurs most often in the winter season
4. Pathophysiology
   a. Bacteria invades epiglottis and surrounding laryngeal area; inflammation and edema rapidly cause airway obstruction
   b. Sudden onset, within a 4 to 12 hour range; medical measures must be instituted rapidly or death may occur
5. Assessment
   a. Assessment findings
      (1) Early signs

    (a) Sore throat

    (b) Fever

    (c) Toxic appearance: sudden onset of fever >102.2° F, respiratory distress, tachypnea, inspiratory stridor, child highly *anxious*, dysphonia (muffled, hoarse voice) present along with drooling

   (2) Other signs indicative of epiglottitis

    (a) Inspiratory stridor

    (b) Absence of a spontaneous cough

    (c) Agitation

    (d) Cherry red and swollen epiglottis

    (e) Red, inflamed oral cavity; drooling

    (f) "Tripod" positioning: while supporting body with hands, child thrusts chin forward and opens mouth in attempt to widen airway

  b. Diagnostic procedures

   (1) Laboratory studies

    (a) Arterial blood gases—decreased pH and PO_2, increased PCO_2—respiratory acidosis

    (b) Throat C&S: identifies causative organism

   (2) Diagnostic studies

    (a) Lateral neck x-ray to confirm diagnosis

    (b) Direct laryngoscopy performed in surgical suite

6. Therapeutic management

 a. Medications

   (1) Analgesics/antipyretics—to reduce fever and throat pain

   (2) Antibiotics—to treat infection

   (3) Immunization: hemophilus type B—to prevent occurrence

 b. Treatments/surgery

   (1) Oxygen therapy—via mask, cannula, or endotracheal tube treats hypoxia; use high humidification to cool airway and decrease swelling

   (2) Endotracheal intubation or tracheostomy, if the child is in severe respiratory distress

   (3) Room humidifier if in the early stage

7. Nursing management

 a. Acute care

   (1) Nursing diagnosis: ineffective airway clearance

(2) Expected outcomes
  (a) Absence of upper airway infectious process
  (b) Return of respiratory state to child's normal parameters
(3) Interventions
  (a) Assess respiratory status, vital signs, nasal flaring, use of accessory muscles, presence of stridor
  (b) Assess breath sounds, skin color changes, attempts to cough
  (c) Observe for signs of increased respiratory distress
  (d) *Avoid visualization* of epiglottis with tongue blade or taking a throat culture to prevent spasm of the epiglottis and airway occlusion
  (e) Provide humidified oxygen
  (f) Maintain in upright position
  (g) Maintain patent airway; assist with emergency procedures; have equipment ready for tracheostomy or intubation
  (h) Provide tracheostomy care as indicated
  (i) Assess hydration status; record intake and output; check for dry mucous membranes, sunken eyes
(4) Nursing diagnosis: anxiety—parents and child
(5) Expected outcomes
  (a) Child and parental anxiety is decreased
  (b) Child's respiratory state returns to or towards the baseline
(6) Interventions
  (a) Assess the level of fear and anxiety of child, parents
  (b) Provide a calm environment
  (c) Remain with child in the acute phase
  (d) Allow the parents to remain with the child
  (e) Inform the parents of the child's status and explain all procedures
  (f) Encourage the parents to express their fears
  b. Home care—refer to the child with pneumonia, p. 162
8. Evaluation
  a. Questions to ask
    (1) What questions do you have about the acute care?
    (2) What will you plan to do for a reoccurrence?

b. Behaviors to observe
   (1) Parents' presence calms and supports child
   (2) Parents' and child's anxious behaviors decrease as respiratory distress is relieved
c. Evaluation of expected outcomes
   (1) Child and family express decreased anxiety as acute stage of disease ends
   (2) Parents remain with the child to provide support
   (3) Child maintains calmer behavior, as air hunger is relieved

C. Laryngotracheobronchitis (LTB)

1. Description: most common form of croup; involves viral infection of larynx, trachea, and bronchi (Table 5-2, p. 178)
2. Etiology: caused by viruses associated with upper respiratory infection—parainfluenza virus, types 1, 2, 3; respiratory syncytial virus; influenza virus: types A1, A2, B; adenovirus; and rhinovirus
3. Incidence
   a. Mainly affects boys; peak age of incidence is 9 to 18 months
   b. Occurs most often in winter months and begins at night
4. Pathophysiology
   a. Viral infection causes mucosal inflammation of the larynx and the trachea; it results in a narrowing of the airway
   b. As the child struggles to move air past the obstruction, negative pressure in the thoracic cavity increases and pulmonary vascular fluid leaks into the interstitial spaces, causing hypoxia
   c. Respiratory acidosis and respiratory failure eventually occur if treatment is delayed
5. Assessment
   a. Assessment findings: four stages of progression in laryngotracheobronchitis (Box 5-1, p. 173)
   b. Diagnostic procedures
      (1) Laboratory studies
         (a) Arterial blood gases—respiratory acidosis— decreased pH and PO_2, increased PCO_2
         (b) Throat culture reveals causative agent
         (c) Complete blood count reveals leukocytosis, if increased WBC >10,000, bacterial infection is present

        (2) Diagnostic studies: chest and neck x-rays rule out epiglottitis

6. Therapeutic management

    a. Medications

        (1) Bronchodilators—"racemic epinephrine" via nebulizer—to relax smooth muscle and relieve stridor; it has a quicker effect for bronchodilation

        (2) Corticosteroids (controversial) for antiinflammatory effect

        (3) Antibiotics if secondary bacterial infection is present

    b. Treatments

        (1) Humidified oxygen or high humidity via vaporizer or tent

        (2) IV fluid therapy for dehydration

        (3) Intubation or tracheostomy if necessary

7. Nursing management

    a. Acute care

        (1) Nursing diagnoses

            (a) Ineffective airway clearance

            (b) Ineffective breathing pattern

        (2) Expected outcomes

            (a) Child's respiratory status returns to child's normal parameters

            (b) Child's breath sounds are clear, with optimum breathing pattern and ventilation

        (3) Interventions

            (a) Assess respirations for a full minute for rate, depth, dyspnea, effort

            (b) Observe for nasal flaring, sternal retractions, inspiratory stridor

            (c) Assess skin color for cyanosis or pallor

            (d) Auscultate breath sounds: rales, crackles, and decreased breath sounds indicate involvement of the bronchi

            (e) Assess cough for persistence, productivity, and characteristic sound

            (f) Administer medications, as ordered, including bronchodilators, antibiotics

            (g) Elevate head of bed to comfort level of child; reposition q 2 hours

            (h) Provide humidification with mist tent or vaporizer

             (i)   Monitor fluid balance

             (j)   Encourage PO intake of clear fluids

             (k) Encourage parents to stay to keep the child calm, which conserves energy for respiratory effort

             (l)   Provide rest periods between procedures

     b. Home care: additional nursing diagnoses

         (1)   Risk for fluid volume deficit

         (2)   Anxiety

         (3)   Fatigue related to work of breathing

         (4)   Interventions: refer to home care of child with pneumonia, p. 162

8. Evaluation

     a. Questions to ask

         (1)   What concerns do you have about your child's breathing problem?

         (2)   What works best to calm your child?

     b. Behaviors to observe

         (1)   Anxiety reduced in parents and child

         (2)   Effective breathing pattern and ventilation return to baseline

     c. Evaluation of expected outcomes

         (1)   Child's respiratory status returns to normal parameters

         (2)   Child's breath sounds are clear

         (3)   Parents' presence calms child and decreases anxiety

III. Infections of the lower respiratory system

  A. Bronchiolitis

     1. Description: inflammation of the smaller bronchioles, caused by a virus and characterized by thick mucus

     2. Etiology

        a. Virus most frequently involved is a respiratory syncytial virus (RSV); others include adenovirus, rhinovirus, and parainfluenza

        b. Transmission is by droplets

     3. Incidence

        a. Frequent cause of hospitalization for infants <1 year of age

        b. Occurs most frequently in the winter and early spring

     4. Pathophysiology

        a. Mucous membranes that line the bronchioles become edematous along with cellular infiltrates and cause obstruction of the smaller airways

      b.   Obstruction of affected airways results in hyperinflation with air trapping occuring

      c.   Hypoxemia is the end result of the hyperinflation of alveoli

  5. Assessment

      a.   Assessment findings

         (1) A history of URI for 1 to 4 days

         (2) Labored respirations

         (3) Hacky, harsh cough

         (4) Difficulty feeding

         (5) Irritability

         (6) Rhonchi; expiratory wheezes

         (7) Low-grade fever: >100° F rectally

      b.   Diagnostic procedures

         (1) Laboratory studies

            (a) Nasal or nasopharyngeal cultures reveal RSV

            (b) CBC—elevated WBC consistent with infection

            (c) Arterial blood gases—decreased pH, PO_2 <60 mm Hg, PCO_2 >45 mm Hg

         (2) Diagnostic studies: chest x-ray—reveals hyperinflation, atelectasis, areas of consolidation, fluid

  6. Therapeutic management: medications

      a.   Antivirals—ribavirin via aerosol during initial days of illness

      b.   Antipyretics—to reduce fever

      c.   Bronchodilators—to relax the smooth muscle of bronchi and bronchioles

  7. Nursing management

      a.   Acute care

         (1) Nursing diagnoses

            (a) Ineffective breathing pattern

            (b) Ineffective airway clearance

            (c) Fatigue

         (2) Interventions: refer to the child with pneumonia

      b.   Home care

         (1) Nursing diagnosis: knowledge deficit

         (2) Interventions and evaluation: refer to the child with pneumonia

B. Pneumonia

  1. Description: inflammation or infection of the pulmonary parenchyma, alveoli

2. Etiology: causative agents that serve as classification of pneumonia
   a. Viruses
   b. Bacteria
   c. Mycoplasmas
   d. Aspiration of foreign substances
3. Incidence
   a. Viral pneumonia occurs more frequently than bacterial pneumonia
   b. Pneumonia occurs more frequently in infancy and early childhood than in the school-age and adolescent periods
4. Pathophysiology
   a. Pattern of the illness depends on the age, causative agent, extent of infection, and systemic reaction to the infection (Table 5-3, p. 179)
   b. May occur as a primary infection or secondary to another illness or infection
5. Assessment
   a. Assessment findings (see Table 5-3, p. 179)
   b. Diagnostic procedures
      (1) Laboratory studies
         (a) CBC: increased WBC >10,000—leukocytosis
         (b) Sputum culture and sensitivity—identifies infectious agent and sensitivity to antimicrobial therapy
         (c) Antistreptolysin-O titer—increased with recent streptococci infection
      (2) Diagnostic studies: chest x-ray—reveals areas of consolidation in one lobe, usually at the bases, or throughout lung, depending on causative agent; if aspiration pneumonia, it is typically in right middle lobe
6. Therapeutic management
   a. Medications
      (1) Antibiotics to treat pneumococcal, streptococcal, staphylococcal pneumonia
      (2) Antipyretics: Tylenol (not ASA) to control fever
   b. Treatment: oxygen therapy with high humidification treats hypoxemia
7. Nursing management
   a. Acute care (also refer to bronchiolitis, p. 161)

        (1) Nursing diagnoses
           (a) Ineffective breathing pattern
           (b) Hyperthermia
           (c) Risk for fluid volume deficit
           (d) Pain/discomfort
        (2) Expected outcomes
           (a) Child recovers without pulmonary complications
           (b) Child's respiratory status return is normal
        (3) Interventions
           (a) Assess vital signs and auscultate lungs q 2 to 4 hours
           (b) Report signs of complications: increased dyspnea, chest pain, cyanosis, abdominal distention, sudden temperature increase
           (c) Inform parents to report changes in sputum, respirations, level of child's comfort
           (d) Instruct parents on medication administration

    b. Home care
        (1) Nursing diagnosis: knowledge deficit
        (2) Expected outcomes
           (a) Parents exhibit knowledge of medication administration and adequate pulmonary toilet
           (b) Child is calm enough to comply with treatments
        (3) Interventions
           (a) Assess parents' and child's knowledge base about pneumonia
           (b) Instruct parents about home care actions: medications and clearing lungs
           (c) Describe the infectious process in the lungs to child in age-appropriate terms

8. Evaluation
    a. Questions to ask
        (1) What concerns you about the acute care of your child?
        (2) What actions might prevent reoccurrence of a pulmonary infection?
    b. Behaviors to observe
        (1) Child's respirations return to within 10% of baseline parameters
        (2) Precautions taken to prevent spread of infection
    c. Evaluation of expected outcomes
        (1) Child recovers without pulmonary complications

(2) Child's temperature remains within 1° of 99.6° F rectally for 24 to 48 hours before discharge

IV. Chronic respiratory conditions of childhood

A. Asthma

1. Description: reversible "reactive" airway disease, characterized by a narrowing of the bronchi and bronchioles; results in lung obstruction and hyperinflation
2. Etiology: asthma attacks are triggered by allergens such as dust, pollen, food, or other causes, including strenuous exercise, weather changes, smoke, viral infections
3. Incidence
   a. Leading chronic lung disorder in children
   b. Majority of children have a first attack before 5 years of age
4. Pathophysiology
   a. Three factors contribute to the findings of obstruction
      (1) Edema of the mucous membranes
      (2) Accumulation of tenacious secretions from the mucous glands
      (3) Smooth muscle spasm of the bronchi and bronchioles
   b. Some children also experience a hypersensitivity component to an asthma attack, which is mediated by IgE
   c. Balance, normally maintained between vagal and sympathetic nerves for smooth muscle tone, is upset by irritants such as dust or smoke
5. Assessment
   a. Assessment findings: symptoms of asthma "attack"
      (1) Audible expiratory wheeze
      (2) Diaphoresis
      (3) Paroxysmal, hacking, and nonproductive cough at onset; becomes rattling and productive for clear sputum
      (4) Restless and apprehensive
      (5) Dyspnea and prolonged expiration
      (6) Nasal flaring
      (7) Intercostal retractions
      (8) Circumoral cyanosis and cyanosis of nailbeds
      (9) Coarse rhonchi
   b. Diagnostic procedures
      (1) Laboratory studies

        (a) Arterial blood gases—reveals decreased pH and PO_2, increased CO_2 as attack progresses

        (b) Sputum culture—reveals presence of eosinophils

        (c) CBC—reveals increased eosinophils in differential

    (2) Diagnostic studies

        (a) Pulmonary function study—reveals decreased tidal volume and vital capacity

        (b) Skin tests—identify specific allergen

        (c) Chest x-ray—reveals hyperinflation, pulmonary infiltrates, and atelectasis

    (3) Complications

        (a) Status asthmaticus

        (b) Chronic emphysema

        (c) Cor pulmonale

        (d) Pneumothorax

        (e) Death if asthma is refractory to therapy

6. Therapeutic management

  a. Medications

    (1) Beta adrenergics—albuterol (Proventil) via inhalation to relax bronchial smooth muscle—bronchodilators used initially to relive acute asthma attacks

    (2) Corticosteroids—suppress hypersensitive reaction and inflammatory response

    (3) Bronchodilators/xanthine: aminophylline, theophylline via IV drip to relax smooth muscle to achieve therapeutic level of 10 to 20 ug/ml; 5 to 15 ug/ml is adequate and considered safer

    (4) Antibiotics—if infection is present

    (5) Antiasthmatic—used prophylactically to manage chronic, severe asthma; cromolyn sodium (Intal) in solution, capsule, or via hand-held meter dose

    (6) Expectorants—to assist with expectoration of excessive mucus; SSKI (potassium iodide)

  b. Treatments

    (1) Oxygen therapy

    (2) Chest physiotherapy

    (3) Injection therapy for hyposensitization

7. Nursing management

  a. Nursing diagnoses

    (1) Acute care

          (a)   Ineffective breathing pattern

          (b)   Ineffective airway clearance

    (2)   Expected outcomes

          (a)   Child breathes easily with normal respiratory effort

          (b)   Child's breath sounds are clear with optimal airflow

          (c)   Child will be able to cough up mucous secretions at least q 1 to 2 hours

    (3)   Interventions

          (a)   Assess respiratory status

          (b)   Auscultate lungs for presence of adventitious breath sounds

          (c)   Assess cough: onset, duration, frequency, productivity, color, and viscosity of sputum

          (d)   Position with head of bed elevated to child's comfort level for breathing

          (e)   Administer pulmonary medications as ordered

          (f)   Assess for signs of aminophylline toxicity; monitor theophylline level >20 µg/ml = toxicity; initial toxicity finding—nausea; later findings—tremors. Note: tachycardia is an expected side effect; a decrease in rate of drip usually decreases HR.

b.   Home care

    (1)   Nursing diagnoses

          (a)   Knowledge deficit

          (b)   Health-seeking behaviors: prevention of asthma attack and secondary infection

    (2)   Expected outcomes

          (a)   Family removes threat of exposure to known allergens

          (b)   Family and child comply with medication regimen

          (c)   Family verbalizes knowledge of the disease process, precipitating factors, symptoms of attack, actions for prevention, and actions to deal with an attack

    (3)   Interventions

          (a)   Assess parents for knowledge of factors related to attacks and measures taken to maintain child's health

          (b)   Teach child and parents how to avoid conditions that precipitate attack; teach methods to

"allergy-proof" the home; may need to have home referral
- (c) Instruct child in breathing exercises with evaluation of effectiveness
- (d) Instruct family in medication administration
- (e) Instruct child to avoid excessive activity and stress
- (f) Teach child correct use of inhalers for technique and early signs for need
- (g) Make referrals to the Asthma and Allergy Foundation of America and the American Lung Association

8. Evaluation
   a. Questions to ask
      (1) How is this attack different from others?
      (2) What concerns or needs do you have about long-term care?
   b. Behaviors to observe
      (1) Child participates in care to the degree of age-appropriate actions
      (2) Parents ask questions or offer actions to make child more comfortable
   c. Evaluation of expected outcomes
      (1) Child avoids exposure to known allergens
      (2) Family complies with prescribed medication regimen
      (3) Family verbalizes understanding of disease process and importance of control of precipitating factors and symptoms of attack

B. **Cystic fibrosis (CF)**
   1. Description: autosomal recessive disorder involving the exocrine glands; characterized by thick, tenacious secretions that affect multiple organs, most commonly
      a. Lungs
      b. Pancreas
      c. Liver
      d. Small intestine
   2. Although the disease is ultimately fatal, the median life expectancy has increased to 27 years of age
   3. Etiology and incidence
      a. The disease affects 1 in 2000 Caucasian infants every year
      b. It is caused by a biochemical defect
      c. When both parents carry the CF gene, 25% of offspring will have CF, 50% will be carriers, and 25% will be normal

4. Pathophysiology
   a. Characteristics of disease process
      (1) Increased viscosity of mucous gland secretions
      (2) Marked elevation of sweat electrolytes: sodium and chloride
      (3) Increased organic and enzymatic constituents of saliva
      (4) Abnormal autonomic nervous system (ANS) function: overactivity of the ANS stimulates cholinergic glands and innervates all exocrine glands
   b. Primary factor responsible for many symptoms of the disease is mechanical obstruction caused by increased viscosity of mucous secretions
   c. Exocrine gland dysfunction affects multiple organ systems (Figure 5-1)
5. Assessment
   a. Assessment findings
      (1) Salty-tasting skin—usually found by parents when they kiss child
      (2) Profuse sweating in warm weather
      (3) Frequent infections
      (4) Dry, nonproductive cough
      (5) Increase in amount and thickness of secretions
      (6) Wheezing, cyanosis
      (7) Digital clubbing from chronic hypoxia
      (8) Increased anterior-posterior diameter of chest
      (9) Steatorrhea (fat in stools); bulky, foul odor to stools
      (10) Thin extremities, muscle wasting
      (11) Failure to thrive
      (12) Meconium ileus (infants)
   b. Diagnostic procedures
      (1) Laboratory studies
         (a) Sweat test—iontophoresis of pilocarpine: a sweat chloride content of >60 mEq is positive for CF
         (b) Stool for fecal fat—reveals impaired fat absorption from pancreatic and liver dysfunction; collected for 72 hours
      (2) Diagnostic studies
         (a) Pulmonary function study—indicates degree of impaired lung function
         (b) Chest x-ray—findings consistent with CF are patchy atelectasis, areas of infiltrates, and bronchopneumonia
         (c) Screening for gene defect for at-risk families

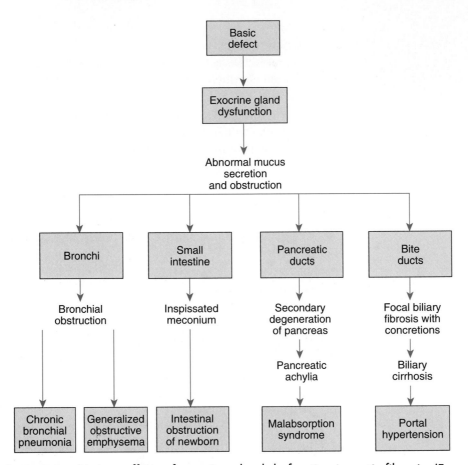

Figure 5-1. Various effects of exocrine gland dysfunction in cystic fibrosis. (From Wong, D: *Whaley and Wong's nursing care of infants and children*, ed 5, St Louis, 1995, Mosby.)

    c. Complications
        (1) Heat prostration
        (2) Bronchiectasis
        (3) Hemoptysis
        (4) Nasal polyps
        (5) Emphysema
        (6) Pneumonia
        (7) Pneumothorax
        (8) Portal hypertension
        (9) Bowel obstruction
      (10) Diabetes mellitus
      (11) Gallstones

      (12) Cirrhosis of the liver

      (13) Cor pulmonale

6. Therapeutic management

   a. Medications

      (1) Bronchodilators/adrenergic agonists—relieve bronchospasm; enable removal of thick secretions; may be given via hand-held nebulizer

      (2) Mucolytics—acetylcysteine (Mucomyst) works on surface tension of mucus to make it more fluid and easier to expectorate

      (3) Pancreatic enzymes—pancrelipase (Viokase) treats pancreatic deficiency; give with meals

      (4) Vitamins—water-miscible forms of A, D, E, and K

      (5) Antibiotics—for prophylactic or infection therapy

      (6) Salt replacement—in warm weather, febrile episodes, increased activity or play

   b. Treatments

      (1) Chest physiotherapy—including postural drainage, chest percussion, vibration, and coughing

      (2) Oxygen therapy—usually for respiratory distress

      (3) Dietary supplementation—usually sodium

      (4) Aerosol therapy—may be routine or PRN

7. Nursing management

   a. Acute care

      (1) Nursing diagnoses

         (a) Ineffective airway clearance

         (b) Ineffective breathing pattern

      (2) Expected outcomes

         (a) Child expectorates mucus with minimal effort

         (b) Child's respiratory status is maintained within 10% of baseline parameters for child

         (c) Child's hydration is maintained by adequate fluid intake and avoidance of hot environments

      (3) Interventions

         (a) Assess for changes in breathing pattern, color and tenacity of mucus, diminished breath sounds, ability to cough and expectorate secretions

         (b) Perform chest physiotherapy before meals

         (c) Assist to cough or suction q 2 hours

         (d) Administer mucolytics, bronchodilators as ordered or indicated by findings

        (4) Nursing diagnosis: altered nutrition—less than body requirements

        (5) Expected outcomes

           (a) Child demonstrates weight gain or no loss of weight

           (b) Child maintains appetite

        (6) Interventions

           (a) Assess child's nutritional status including height and weight

           (b) Administer pancreatic enzyme immediately before meals and snacks

           (c) Provide salt, especially during hot weather or excessive play

           (d) Teach parents that they can mix oral enzyme with pureed applesauce and administer with a spoon

    b. Home care

        (1) Nursing diagnosis: altered family processes

        (2) Expected outcomes

           (a) Family adjusts to changes in lifestyle

           (b) Family develops positive coping strategies

           (c) Family receives support from appropriate community agencies

        (3) Interventions

           (a) Assist in identifying and using effective coping strategies on a daily basis

           (b) Refer to counseling services, local support agencies for CF, and the CF Foundation

           (c) Encourage parents to express fears and concerns

        (4) Other nursing diagnoses

           (a) Risk for infection

           (b) Altered growth and development

           (c) Risk for activity intolerance

8. Evaluation

    a. Questions to ask

        (1) What needs do you have for home care?

        (2) How are you coping with the stress of daily care of the child?

        (3) What kind of help will decrease your stress or help your child's physical or emotional status?

    b. Behaviors to observe
        (1) Family adheres to prescribed medical regimen including follow-up care
        (2) Family seeks support from appropriate agencies
    c. Evaluation of expected outcomes
        (1) Child maintains respiratory status within 10% of baseline parameters
        (2) Child able to cough up thick mucous secretions
        (3) Child remains free of infection and maintains weight above the 25th percentile for stature

---

Box 5-1. Progression of Findings in Laryngotracheobronchitis

Stage I

Fear
Hoarseness
Croupy cough
Inspiratory stridor when disturbed

Stage II

Continuous respiratory stridor
Lower rib retraction
Retraction of soft tissue of neck
Use of accessory muscles of respiration
Labored respiration

Stage III

Signs of anoxia and carbon dioxide retention
Restlessness
Anxiety
Pallor
Sweating
Rapid respiration

Stage IV

Intermittent cyanosis
Permanent cyanosis
Cessation of breathing

As described by Forbes from Krugman, S., and others: *Infectious diseases of children*, St Louis, 1985, Mosby.

Table 5-1. Commonly Used Pulmonary Medications for Children

Classification	Medication	Indications	Route and Dosage	Side Effects	Nursing Implications
Broncho-dilator	Generic: aminophyllin (IV) theophylline (PO) Trade: Somophyllin	Bronchial asthma Chronic bronchitis Emphysema	IV (Maintenance) >24 days 1.9 mg/kg q 12 hr 1-9 years: 1 mg/kg/hr 9-12 years: 0.9 mg/kg/hr 12-16 years: 0.6 mg/kg/hr PO 1-9 years: 20 mg/kg/ day 9-16 years: 16 mg/kg/ day	CNS: Drowsiness, lethargy, fatigue, agitation, *tremors GI: Anorexia, *nausea, vomiting Hepatic: Jaundice, hepatitis GU: Urinary retention Integumentary: Rash, erythema CV: Prolonged PR intervals, postural hypotension, tachycardia, hypertension	Administer PO with food to decrease GI upset Assess respiratory status Monitor daily serum drug levels (10-20 mcg/ml); toxicity >20 mcg/ml or if symptoms persist Parent education: Administer at same time daily to maintain levels Report any CNS, cardiac, or GI side effects to physician

*Common toxic signs

Classification	Drug	Use	Dosage	Side Effects	Nursing Considerations
Beta-adrenergic Selective B$_2$ agonist	Generic: metaproterenol Trade: Alupent	Bronchial asthma Bronchospasm	PO *<6 years:* 1.3-2.6 mg/kg/day *6-9 years:* 10 mg qid *>9 years:* 20 mg tid or qid Aerosol 2-3 inhalations q 3-4 hrs maximum 12 inhalations/day	*CNS:* Tachycardia, tremors, dysrhythmia *GI:* Nausea, vomiting *Other:* Insomnia	Assess respiratory status Do not crush tablet Shake canister well; wait 2 minutes before second inhalation *Parent education:* Teach proper usage and care of inhaler or spacer Have child return demonstrate use of inhaler Should not be used more frequently than prescribed
B$_2$ agonist	Generic: terbutaline Trade: Brethine	Asthma Emphysema	PO *>12 years:* 0.05 mg/kg dose tid Aerosol Two inhalations (400 mcg) q 4-6 hr	*CNS:* Nervousness, lethargy, headache *CV:* Palpitations, tachycardia, dysrhythmias *GI:* Nausea, vomiting	Assess respiratory status and baseline heart rate Do not crush time-release tablets Mix regular tablets with small amounts of food or fluid

Continued.

Table 5-1. Commonly Used Pulmonary Medications for Children—cont'd

Classification	Medication	Indications	Route and Dosage	Side Effects	Nursing Implications
B$_2$ agonist				*Sensory:* Dry nose and mouth, tinnitus	*Parent education:* Teach correct inhalation technique Do not exceed dosage Do not use with other inhalants
Expectorants	Generic: guaifenesin Trade: Robitussin DM	Productive cough	PO *2-5 years:* 50-100 mg q hr (not to exceed 600 mg/day) *6-11 years:* 100-200 mg q hr (not to exceed 1.2 g/day)	*CNS:* Drowsiness *GI:* Nausea, vomiting, diarrhea	Assess respiratory status, cough frequency Increase fluid intake; maintain hydration Monitor BP Provide cool mist vaporizer

Classification	Generic/Trade	Indications	Dosage	Side Effects	Nursing Considerations
	Generic: terpin hydrate Trade: Terphan	Cough	PO *1-4 years:* 20-25 mg tid-qid *5-9 years:* 40-45 mg tid-qid *10-12 years:* 85 mg tid-qid	*GI:* Nausea, vomiting	Assess cough Maintain hydration Children <12 years should only be given medication under physician's care
Mucolytic	Generic: acetylcysteine Trade: Mucomyst	Cystic fibrosis Bronchitis Pneumonia Emphysema Acetaminophen overdosage	Inhalation 3-5 ml of 20% solution 6-10 ml of 10% solution 3-4 times per day	*CNS:* Drowsiness *GI:* Nausea, vomiting doses, stomatitis *Respiratory:* Bronchospasm *Integumentary:* Urticaria	Assess cough and type of mucous secretions Have a child cough before nebulization Nebulized drug should be inhaled from face mask or tent
			PO only for acetaminophen overdosage: 70 mg/kg dose q 4 hr × 17 doses (initial doses 140 mg/kg)		

From Wong, D: *Whaley and Wong's nursing care of infants and children*, ed 5, St Louis, 1995, Mosby.

Table 5-2. Comparison of Croup Syndromes

Factors	Acute Epiglottitis (Supraglottitis)	Acute Laryngo-tracheobronchitis (LTB)	Acute Spasmodic Laryngitis (Spasmodic Croup)	Acute Tracheitis
Age group affected	1 to 8 years	3 months to 8 years	3 months to 3 years	1 month to 6 years
Etiologic agent	Bacterial, usually *H. influenzae*	Viral	Viral with allergic component	Bacterial, usually *S. aureus*
Onset	Rapidly progressive	Slowly progressive	Sudden; at night	Moderately progressive
Major symptoms	Dysphagia Stridor aggravated when supine Drooling High fever Toxic Rapid pulse and respirations	URI Stridor Brassy cough Hoarseness Dyspnea Restlessness Irritability Low-grade fever Nontoxic	URI Croupy cough Stridor Hoarseness Dyspnea Restlessness Symptoms waken child Symptoms disappear during day Tends to recur	URI Croupy cough Stridor Purulent secretions High fever No response to LTB therapy
Treatment	Antibiotics Airway protection	Humidity Racemic epinephrine	Humidity	Antibiotics

From Wong, D: *Whaley and Wong's nursing care of infants and children*, ed 5, St Louis, 1995, Mosby.

Table 5-3. Comparison of Types of Pneumonia in Children Based on Etiologic Agents

Type	Etiologic Agents	Age Group Affected	Assessment Findings	Treatments
Viral pneumonia	RSV Influenza Parainfluenza Rhinovirus Adenovirus	All age groups	Mild to high fever Cough Rhonchi, crackles	Symptomatic Fluids if dehydration
Bacterial pneumonia	Staphyloccocus pneumonia Group A streptococcus Staphyloccus H. influenza	All age groups 3 months to 5 years: pneumococcal and H. influenza >5 years: pneumococcal	Abdominal pain Chest pain Cough Adventitious breath sounds Irritability; poor feeding Spike in temperature	Antibiotic therapy Bed rest Antipyretics for fever PO fluids Mist tent
Primary atypical pneumonia	(Myeoplasma) pneumonia	5 to 12 years	Fever, chills Headache, malaise, anoretic Sore throat Dry, hacking cough Myalgia—aching muscles	Symptomatic
Aspiration pneumonia	Food, fluids Vitamins Nasopharyngeal secretions Hydrocarbons	Infants, young children	Coughing Choking Dyspnea Fever Typically found in right middle lobe, since right bronchi is most vertical	Oxygen therapy Hydration Treatment of secondary infection Note: vomiting is contraindicated in hydrocarbon pneumonia

From Wong, D: *Whaley and Wong's nursing care of infants and children*, ed 5, St Louis, 1995, Mosby.

REVIEW QUESTIONS

1. A 10-year-old boy with a severe asthma attack is brought to the emergency department by his parents. Considering the child's diagnosis, the child is most likely to have which of these findings?
   a. Hacking, nonproductive cough
   b. Itching at base of neck or upper back
   c. Shortness of breath, prolonged expiratory phase
   d. Mild, inspiratory wheezing

2. Eight-year-old Gina is admitted to the pediatric unit with a respiratory infection. She was diagnosed with cystic fibrosis as an infant. The physician orders all of the following medications for Gina. Which one should the nurse question?
   a. Bronchodilator
   b. Antitussive
   c. Mucolytic agent
   d. Pancreatic enzyme

3. With the medical diagnosis of severe asthma, which of these nursing diagnoses would be most appropriate?
   a. Altered family processes
   b. Body-image disturbance
   c. Ineffective breathing pattern
   d. Risk for infection

4. Following a myringotomy, which intervention would facilitate drainage from the ear?
   a. Apply a gauze pack tightly to the affected ear
   b. Apply a warm pack to the affected ear
   c. Position the child on the affected side
   d. Position the child in a prone position

5. Following a tonsillectomy, a child grows increasingly restless. The nurse assesses the child to find a pulse rate of 120 and frequent swallowing. Based on these findings, the nurse should suspect the client has which of these conditions?
   a. Airway obstruction
   b. Hemorrhage
   c. Infection
   d. Usual signs following this surgery

6. A 3-year-old is brought to the emergency department with the following symptoms: fever, restlessness, and drooling. No coughing is observed. Based on these findings, the nurse should
   a. Continuously monitor airway status
   b. Examine the throat with tongue depressor
   c. Take a throat culture
   d. Prepare antibiotics for infusion

7. A mother states that her child experienced shortness of breath following lunch at a local fast food restaurant. She states that the following foods were eaten. The one most likely to have caused an allergic reaction is
   a. Chocolate shake
   b. Salad
   c. Turkey sandwich
   d. Baked potato

8. An emergency department nurse is assessing a 5-year-old experiencing an acute asthma attack. Which one of these findings should be reported immediately?
   a. Absence of wheezing
   b. Cyanosis
   c. Nonproductive cough
   d. Prolonged expiratory phase

9. The assessment of a child brought to the emergency department reveals dyspnea, moderate fever, sore throat, and drooling. The mother describes the onset of the symptoms as "sudden." The nurse should suspect that the child has which of these conditions?
   a. Asthma
   b. Croup
   c. Epiglottitis
   d. Bronchiolitis

10. The parent of a 10-year-old with cystic fibrosis receives instructions regarding chest physiotherapy. Which statement by the parent indicates the need for further teaching?
   a. "I'll start physiotherapy with a nebulizer treatment"
   b. "I'll plan to do chest physiotherapy after breakfast"
   c. "I plan to do postural drainage, percussion, and vibration"
   d. "Chest physiotherapy must be done several times daily"

11. A child is admitted to the pediatric unit, and intravenous therapy is started. Administration of aminophylline has been ordered. A priority nursing action during the aminophylline infusion is to
    a. Assess capillary refill
    b. Ensure adequate fluid intake
    c. Monitor vital signs
    d. Provide diversional activity

12. Which of the following statements is accurate regarding the mode of transmission for autosomal recessive disorders such as cystic fibrosis (CF)?
    a. Both parents must have the disease to have a child with CF
    b. There is a 75% chance with each pregnancy that the child will have CF
    c. Both parents must be carriers of the trait in order for the child to have the disease
    d. There is a 50% chance with each pregnancy that the child will not have CF

ANSWERS, RATIONALES, AND TEST-TAKING TIPS

Rationales	Test-Taking Tips

1. **Correct answer: c**

    A child with a severe asthma attack is short of breath and tries to breathe more deeply; the expiratory phase becomes prolonged and is accompanied by audible (heard without a stethoscope) wheezing. Asthma attacks begin with a hacking, nonproductive cough. Itching at the base of the neck or over the upper back is observed in the prodromal phase. Wheezing can occur on inspiration or expiration; however, in severe asthma the wheezing would be more than "mild."

    Key words in the stem are "severe asthma attack." Thus, shortness of breath would be characteristic.

2. **Correct answer: b**

    A medication that inhibits coughing should be questioned. The increased viscosity of respiratory secretions in cystic fibrosis contributes to the risk of infection. Coughing moves secretions for expectoration and therefore decreases the risk of infection. The medications in options *a, c,* and *d* would not be questioned. Bronchodilators are usually ordered via nebulizer to open the bronchi for easier breathing and expectoration. Mucolytic agents are used to decrease

    Cystic fibrosis affects the systems that have exocrine secretions—lungs, liver, gastrointestinal tract, pancreas. The secretions become very thick and tend to result in obstructions.

the viscosity of mucous secretions or relieve meconium ileus. Pancreatic enzymes are administered with meals and snacks to ensure that digestive enzymes are mixed with food in the duodenum.

3. Correct answer: c

This nursing diagnosis is most appropriate for the situation of bronchospasm and the need to improve ventilatory capacity. In Maslow's hierarchy of needs, the need for air takes top priority over infection or any of the given psychosocial needs. The items in options *a* and *b* are psychosocial concerns appropriate to the care plan of the child with asthma. Option *d* describes a "potential" or risk problem; there are no data to support that infection is an actual problem. The child with asthma should be protected from respiratory infections, which can trigger an asthma attack.

Eliminate responses *a* and *b,* since they are psychosocial and there is not data to support them as diagnoses. Between *c* and *d*, both physiologic needs, select response *c,* since airway, breathing, and circulation are priorities over other needs. Another approach, if you have no idea of the correct response, is to simply match up the problem, "severe asthma," with a similar word or item in one of the responses, response *c*— "breathing." Select response *c*.

4. Correct answer: c

Being on the affected side facilitates drainage of the exudate from the affected ear. A gauze pack should be applied loosely to allow accumulated drainage to flow out of the ear and onto the gauze. Local dry heat such

The words that make two responses incorrect are: in response *a*, "tightly," and in response *b*, "warm pad." Between response *c* and *d,* use common sense: to drain something it is put downward. Select response *c*.

as a hot water bottle may decrease the pain but does not facilitate drainage. Warm soaks would be contraindicated, since the moistness may flow into the ear and cause further infection. The prone position is not an effective action to facilitate drainage from the ear.

5. Correct answer: b

The most obvious early sign of bleeding is a client's frequent swallowing of blood trickling down the throat. Airway obstruction after a tonsillectomy is indicated by findings of upper airway obstruction such as inspiratory stridor or sternal retractions from the increased effort needed to pull air through an edematous upper airway. The findings in option *c* are not consistent with infection. Option *d* is a false statement. Discomfort in swallowing is expected after this surgery.

Remember that a first sign of bleeding is an increased heart rate, usually defined as a sustained increase in heart rate of 20 beats per minute over the baseline rate.

6. Correct answer: a

Three clinical observations have been known to predict epiglottitis: absence of a spontaneous cough, presence of drooling from edema and difficulty in swallowing, and agitation from hypoxia. Continuous monitoring of respiratory status is a priority. When epiglottitis is suspected,

Given the choices, use the principles of basic life support (BLS): airway, breathing and circulation (ABCs) to select response *a*, an intervention related to airway and breathing.

nurses should not attempt to visualize the epiglottis or take a throat culture. In option *d,* there are not enough data in the stem to select this response.

7. **Correct answer: a**

Chocolate is a hyperallergenic food source. Some foods can cause asthma-type reactions; parents need to be advised to eliminate foods known to provoke symptoms. The foods in options *b, c,* and *d* are not known to cause allergic reactions.

Milk products and chocolate in products more commonly cause reactions in children and adults. Pulmonary, gastrointestinal, and neurological (headache) findings are reported.

8. **Correct answer: a**

The absence of wheezing is an ominous sign that indicates respiratory failure from the collapse of the bronchioles. In options *b, c,* and *d* the findings are associated with asthma attacks.

Contrary to common thought, the sudden absence of wheezing in acute asthma attacks indicates a respiratory emergency. The nurse should stay with the client and call for help.

9. **Correct answer: c**

The child diagnosed with epiglottitis usually awakens with complaints of a sore throat. The child will also have a fever. Drooling is common because of the pain associated with swallowing, which is not done with the usual frequency, and the excess secretions from the inflammation. In option *a* the findings consistent with asthma are wheezing, shortness of breath, and

If you have no idea of the correct answer, cluster responses *a, b,* and *d* under lower respiratory tract problems. Select option *c* which is an upper respiratory tract problem. Recall tip: Drooling in children with respiratory distress is a classic sign of epiglottitis.

prolonged expiration. In option *b* the findings consistent with croup are croupy cough and inspiratory stridor. In option *d* the findings consistent with bronchiolitis are tachypnea, paroxysmal cough, and wheezing.

10. Correct answer: b

Chest physiotherapy is generally performed before meals to minimize the chance of vomiting. The responses in *a, c,* and *d* indicate adequate knowledge. Bronchodilator medications delivered in aerosol via a nebulizer help open or dilate the bronchi for easier expectoration and breathing. Chest physiotherapy includes the use of postural drainage in combination with adjunct techniques of percussion and vibration, which are believed to enhance the removal of mucus from the airway. Chest physiotherapy is usually performed twice daily and more frequently if the child experiences a respiratory infection.

The first step should be to reread the question. Note that the question is to identify a statement for "the need for further teaching"—an incorrect statement. Next, apply this general principle: procedures are typically not done after meals. This information will guide you to select response *b*.

11. Correct answer: c

Pulse, respiration, and BP are taken and recorded every 5 minutes during rapid infusion and every 15 minutes for at least an hour after the drug has been absorbed; extreme

If you have no idea of a correct answer, use the airway, breathing and circulation (ABCs) approach. Option *c* is the only option that includes respiratory concerns.

sustained tachycardia, (e.g., >140) may be an early sign of toxicity. A slight increase in the heart rate is expected. Option *a* is not an essential observation during an aminophylline infusion. Checking capillary refill, the arterial circulation, is a priority after cast application to an extremity. Fluids are important but not the priority; the child should receive sufficient fluids either orally or intravenously to replace losses from diaphoresis and hyperventilation. Option *d* is an important consideration for the pediatric client; however, it is not the priority action during aminophylline infusion.

12. Correct answer: c

The affected child inherits the defective gene from both parents; the parents must be carriers of the trait. There is a 1:4 ratio or 25% chance with each pregnancy that the child will have cystic fibrosis. There is a 25% chance the child will be unaffected.

The approach to use here is "go with what you know" plus common sense. Eliminate options *b* and *d* since you can recall exact percentages. In deciding between options *a* and *c,* it is more logical to have a trait than to have a disease for the transmission of a disease.

Nursing Care of Children with Gastrointestinal Disorders

STUDY OUTCOMES

After completing this chapter, the reader will be able to do the following:

▼ List common diagnostic and laboratory tests used to evaluate gastrointestinal function.

▼ Describe the physiological characteristics of young children that predispose them to fluid imbalances.

▼ Differentiate among various types of dehydration.

▼ Describe the pathophysiology and the assessment findings of obstructive disorders: pyloric stenosis, intussusception.

▼ Describe the nursing management of the pediatric obstructive disorders: pyloric stenosis, intussusception.

▼ Outline the major principles of diet therapy for a child with celiac disease.

▼ Discuss the management and nursing considerations for a child with an inflammatory disorder: appendicitis.

▼ Develop a teaching plan for parents to prevent the ingestion of a foreign substance by children.

KEY TERMS

Ascites	Abnormal intraperitoneal accumulation of a fluid containing large amounts of protein and electrolytes; may be detectable when more than 500 ml of fluid has accumulated.
Bruit	Abnormal sound or murmur heard while auscultating a carotid artery, organ, or gland.
Hernia	Protrusion of an organ through an abnormal opening in the muscle wall of the cavity that surrounds it.
Malabsorption	Impaired absorption of nutrients from the gastrointestinal tract.
McBurney's point	Site of extreme sensitivity in acute appendicitis; situated in the normal area of the appendix about 2 inches from the right anterior superior spine of the ileum on a line between that spine and the umbilicus.
Pica	Craving to eat substances that are not foods.
Rebound tenderness	Sign of inflammation of the peritoneum in which pain is elicited by the sudden release of a hand pressing on the abdomen; common finding in peritonitis and appendicitis.
Stricture	Abnormal temporary or permanent narrowing of the lumen of a hollow organ such as the esophagus, pylorus of the stomach, ureter, or urethra caused by inflammation, external pressure, or scarring.

CONTENT REVIEW

I. **The Gastrointestinal (GI) system**
   A. **Review of structure and function**
      1. Anatomy
         a. GI system includes: mouth, pharynx, esophagus, stomach, duodenum, jejunum and ileum, colon (ascending, transverse, descending, and sigmoid), rectum, and anus, as well as the accessory organs of the liver, gallbladder, and pancreas
         b. Ingestion, digestion, and absorption of nutrients by the GI tract are essential for life
         c. Structure of GI wall throughout the system is similar and contains four layers

        (1) Mucosa—contains connective tissue, lymphatic and blood capillaries, and two muscle layers

        (2) Submucosa—consists of connective tissue, lymphatic and blood vessels, and a nerve-fiber complex

        (3) Muscularis—consists of two muscle layers and a nerve-fiber complex

        (4) Serosa—contains connective tissue covered by a single layer of mesothelial cells

    d. The sympathetic and parasympathetic branches of the autonomic nervous system enter the GI tract and synapse with two major plexuses to influence motor and secretory activity

        (1) Sympathetic effect: decreased peristalsis and secretions from the mucous membrane

        (2) Parasympathetic effect: maintenance of peristalsis and mucous membrane secretions

    e. Enzymes

        (1) Pancreatic: trypsin, lipase, and amylase—stimulated by proteins, fats, and carbohydrates

        (2) Gallbladder: bile—stimulated by fat

2. GI development

    a. In embryonic development, the branchial arches, foregut, midgut, and hindgut give rise to the GI tract

    b. During the fourth week of gestation, the foregut, midgut, and hindgut are formed when the dorsal portion of the yolk sac is incorporated into the embryo

    c. Oral cavity, developed from branchial arches, develops early in fourth week of gestation

3. Major functions

    a. Assists in maintaining fluid and electrolyte and acid/base balance

    b. Processes and absorbs nutrients to maintain metabolism and support growth and development

    c. Excretes waste products from the digestive processes

B. Assessment

   1. Health history

    a. General

        (1) Diet

           (a) Typical 24-hour food intake

           (b) Food preferences and dislikes

           (c) Food intolerances

           (d) Religious, cultural food preferences

    (e) Weight gain or loss; over what period of time

    (f) Pica—craving to ingest nonfood substances such as clay, chalk, or starch

   (2) Medications: use and frequency of use for

    (a) Laxatives, stool softeners, antidiarrheal agents

    (b) Antiemetics, antacids

    (c) Aspirin, acetaminophen, nonsteroid antiinflammatories

    (d) Antibiotics

   (3) Activity

    (a) Recent stressful events

    (b) Exposure to infectious diseases

    (c) Recent travel history

  b. Present condition

   (1) Abdominal discomfort, distention

   (2) Indigestion

   (3) Nausea

   (4) Vomiting: describe character, amount, and frequency

   (5) Diarrhea: describe character, amount, and frequency

   (6) Constipation: toilet-training methods

  c. History

   (1) GI disorder: intestinal obstruction

   (2) Abdominal injury or surgery

  d. Family history

   (1) Colon cancer

   (2) Malabsorption syndrome

   (3) Hirschprung disease

 2. Physical examination

  a. Abdomen—follow listed sequence of assessment

   (1) Inspection

    (a) Surface characteristics

    (b) Presence of umbilical hernia

    (c) Contour—infant, toddler: rounded "pot belly"

    (d) Surface motion—peristalsis not usually visible

    (e) Distention

   (2) Auscultation

    (a) Presence of bowel sounds

    (b) Vascular sounds—venous hums, bruits should not be heard

   (3) Percussion

    (a) Tone—children's abdomens sound louder in tympanic tones

(b) Liver span
    (i) 6-month-old: 2.4 to 2.8 cm
    (ii) 5-year-old: 7 cm
    (iii) 12-year-old: 9 cm
    (iv) 16-year-old: 6 to 12 cm
(4) Palpation
    (a) Tenderness, firmness, softness
    (b) Assess all four quadrants
    (c) Organs: spleen, kidney, bladder
    (d) If suspicious of neoplasm, especially near kidney, limit manipulation of mass
b. Anal/rectal region: surface characteristics and tenderness
3. Related laboratory and diagnostic studies (Table 6-1, p. 217)

C. **Commonly used GI medications for children (Table 6-2, pp. 218-223)**

II. Major concepts of fluid and electrolyte balance

A. **Distribution of body fluids**
1. Total body water comprises 65% to 85% of body weight in infants and children
2. Body water is divided into two major fluid compartments
    a. Extracellular fluid (ECF)—contained outside of cell walls; infants and children have a greater proportion of water here; subdivided into
        (1) interstitial—between cells
        (2) intravascular—plasma in vascular bed
    b. Intracellular fluid (ICF)—contained within cell walls; therefore, fluid is more protected within this less-exposed environment
3. Infants and children are more vulnerable to fluid volume deficit because a greater amount of their body water is in the ECF compartment, which offers less protection to fluid losses; also, organs that conserve water are immature, especially the kidneys
4. Children and infants have a greater free water turnover than adults from their
    a. Increased basal metabolic rate with increased evaporative losses
    b. Elevated resting respiratory rate that adds to their fluid losses

B. Acid-base balance
1. Dependent on the following
   a. Chemical buffers
   b. Renal and respiratory system involvement
   c. 20:1 ratio of base bicarbonate to carbonic acid
   d. Dilution of strong acids and bases in blood
2. Acids donate H^+ ions; bases are alkaline substances that readily accept H^+ ions
3. Imbalances of acid-base in extracellular fluids
   a. Respiratory acidosis from carbonic acid excess, e.g., asthma, pneumonia
   b. Respiratory alkalosis from a carbonic acid deficit, e.g., hyperventilation in fever and encephalitis
   c. Metabolic acidosis from a base bicarbonate deficit, e.g., diabetic acidosis, decreased food intake, severe dehydration, severe diarrhea
   d. Metabolic alkalosis from a base bicarbonate excess, e.g., vomiting, excessive gastric tube losses

C. Dehydration in infants and children
1. Most common fluid and electrolyte imbalance in children
2. Losses of extracellular fluid and electrolytes caused by
   a. Vomiting
   b. Diarrhea
   c. Burns
   d. Malnutrition
   e. Diaphoresis
   f. Decreased fluid intake
3. Classification of dehydration (Table 6-3, p. 224)
   a. Isotonic dehydration
   b. Hypotonic dehydration
   c. Hypertonic dehydration
4. Degree of dehydration is determined by the percentage of fluid loss from preillness to current illness state
   a. Mild: 5% weight loss
   b. Moderate: 10% weight loss
   c. Severe: 15% weight loss
5. More accurate classification involves the loss of milliliters per kilogram of body weight over 48 hours or less
   a. Mild: <50 ml/kg
   b. Moderate: 50 to 90 ml/kg
   c. Severe: >100 ml/kg

6. Signs of dehydration
   a. Weight loss
   b. Decreased urine output, increased specific gravity
   c. Dry mucous membranes
   d. Sunken anterior fontanel
   e. Prolonged capillary refill time
   f. Absence of tears
   g. Tachycardia
   h. Hemoconcentration: increased H&H
   i. Decrease in skin turgor

III. Conditions that produce fluid and electrolyte imbalance

A. Vomiting
   1. Definition: forceful expulsion of stomach contents
   2. Common findings of childhood are associated with the following conditions
      a. Allergic reaction
      b. Infection
      c. Overfeeding
      d. Toxin exposure
      e. Infection: urinary and respiratory tract
      f. CNS disorders
      g. Side effect of drugs
      h. Obstructive disorders such as pyloric stenosis and intussusception
   3. The following findings often accompany vomiting
      a. Nausea
      b. Diarrhea
      c. Abdominal cramping; pain
      d. Headache
   4. Careful assessment of the following findings are useful in evaluating the cause of vomiting
      a. Character of vomitus
      b. Frequency and persistence
      c. Amount
      d. Force—projectile typical of pyloric stenosis or increased intracranial pressure
   5. Metabolic alkalosis and dehydration may develop with prolonged, severe vomiting
   6. Home management of short-term vomiting in older children is possible; use of BRAT diet: bananas, rice cereal, applesauce, and toast until nausea/vomiting subside

   7. Hospitalization is necessary when signs of dehydration, blood in vomitus, forceful vomiting, or abdominal pain are present
   8. Nursing diagnoses
       a. Fluid volume deficit
       b. Altered nutrition: less than body requirements

B. **Diarrhea**
    1. Definition: accelerated excretion of intestinal contents; may be acute or chronic in nature
    2. Acute diarrhea associated with the following
        a. Gastroenteritis
        b. Dietary indiscretions: overfeeding, excess sugar or fat in formula; sensitivities to cow's milk, eggs, wheat, nuts, shellfish, glutens
        c. Antibiotic use: medications such as ampicillin and tetracycline cause decreased glucose absorption and disaccharidase activity; also, antibiotic use allows for the overgrowth of a bacterium that causes pseudomembranous colitis
        d. Other illnesses: urinary or respiratory tract infections
    3. Chronic nonspecific diarrhea (CNSD) is the most common cause of protracted diarrhea in young children, especially in the toddler age group
        a. Caused by decreased transit time in alimentary tract
        b. Factors associated with CNSD
            (1) Food intolerance
            (2) Excessive fluid intake
            (3) Protein or carbohydrate intolerance
            (4) Drug administration
    4. Other conditions associated with chronic diarrhea
        a. Cystic fibrosis
        b. Parasitic infections
    5. Wide variety of stooling patterns occur in infants and children; the following criteria must be present to identify diarrhea
        a. Increased frequency of stools
        b. Watery consistency
        c. Stool color becomes green
    6. Complications of acute and chronic diarrhea
        a. Dehydration
        b. Metabolic acidosis
        c. Malnutrition
    7. Treatment of diarrhea includes
        a. Placing bowel at rest by keeping the child NPO

       b. Fluid and electrolyte replacement; *no potassium should be added to intravenous solution until child has voided; this ensures adequate renal function*

       c. Elimination of underlying cause

    8. Nursing diagnoses

       a. Fluid volume deficit

       b. Altered nutrition: less than body requirements

C. **Acute gastroenteritis (GE) (Table 6-4, pp. 225-226)**

    1. Definition: inflammation of stomach and intestines, which may be acute or chronic

    2. Caused by various organisms, allergies, disease processes, contaminated foods

    3. Infectious GE is a term used when the diarrhea is caused by bacteria or virus

IV. Congenital defects: cleft lip and palate

A. **Description: failure of soft tissue and/or bony structure to fuse during embryonic development; may occur separately or together and involve one or both sides of the palate's midline**

B. **Etiology: caused by fetal insult; teratogenic factors include**

    1. Drugs

    2. Exposure to radiation

    3. Exposure to rubella virus

    4. Chromosomal abnormalities

C. **Incidence**

    1. Often occur with other congenital anomalies such as spina bifida

    2. Congenital defects occur mostly in Caucasian and Japanese populations

D. **Pathophysiology**

    1. Lip: maxillary prominence fails to fuse with medial nasal prominence between seventh and eighth week of intrauterine life

    2. Palate: failure of maxillary bone plate to close during seventh to twelfth weeks of intrauterine life

    3. Cleft lip and palate may occur as isolated defect or in combination with each other

E. **Assessment**

    1. Clefts of lip: unilateral or bilateral; extent varies from a slight notch in the vermillion border to a complete separation from the floor of the nose

    2. Cleft palate: unilateral or bilateral; varying degree for the extent of palate involvement that is evident upon visual inspection

F. Therapeutic management

    1. Surgery: plastic surgical correction of cleft lip during first 3 months of life; palate correction done either at 12 or 18 months, before speech habits are established, or delayed until 4 years of age; corrections often require several stages

    2. Medications: analgesics (narcotic, nonnarcotic) to control postoperative pain

    3. Feeding devices: use of soft, elongated lambs' nipples; Brecht feeder (aspeto syringe with rubber tubing attached) is useful for infants with a large cleft palate

    4. Speech therapy: ongoing

G. Nursing management

    1. Preoperative care

       a. Nursing diagnosis: altered nutrition—less than body requirements

       b. Expected outcome: parents demonstrate effective feeding technique

       c. Interventions

          (1) Assess infant's feeding requirements

          (2) Assess nature of defect and its impact on feeding

          (3) Monitor respiratory status and ability to suck during feeding

          (4) Encourage breast feeding if appropriate

          (5) Initiate feeding with special devices, as required: Brecht feeder, lambs' nipple

          (6) Feed small amounts gradually

          (7) Burp frequently: every 15 to 30 cc

          (8) Demonstrate special feeding or suctioning techniques to parents

          (9) Support parents in their efforts

    2. Postoperative care

       a. Nursing diagnosis: risk for injury, infection

       b. Expected outcome: suture line remains clean and free of trauma and infection

       c. Interventions

          (1) Assess suture line for drainage, crusting, signs of infection

          (2) Cleft lip repair: cleanse lip suture line after feeding and as ordered; use cotton-tipped applicator

moistened with saline or other solution as preferred by surgeon

(3) Position the infant on back or on side; avoid the abdomen (prone) to prevent rubbing of surgical site on mattress

(4) Maintain lip protective device—Logan bow on operative site

(5) Restrain with soft elbow or jacket restraints; remove, one at a time, periodically to perform range of motion exercises

(6) Avoid contact with sharp objects, straws, or forks near surgical site

(7) Anticipate child's needs to prevent crying

(8) Feed with cup, wide bowl or soup spoon—not a regular spoon; if palate repaired: avoid inserting spoon into mouth, which may disrupt sutures

(9) Avoid the use of oral suction or placing objects in mouth such as a tongue depressor, oral thermometer

(10) Prevent sucking: no pacifiers or use of straws for oral fluid intake

   3. Additional nursing diagnoses

     a. Ineffective airway clearance

     b. Anxiety

     c. Ineffective family coping

H. Evaluation

   1. Absence of trauma and infection at incision site

   2. Patent airway maintained without pulmonary aspiration

   3. Parents provide appropriate feeding techniques and incision care

V. Gastric ingestion of foreign substances

A. Pica: habitual, purposeful act of craving for and ingestion of nonfood substances such as dirt, chalk, clay, starch, paint chips, crayons

   1. Certain forms are associated with mineral deficiency. Example: eating chalk is linked to calcium deficiency.

   2. Sometimes pica is a factor in lead poisoning; however, most cases of lead poisoning are associated with child's instinctual behavior to explore with the mouth

B. Poisonings—common accidental ingestions
(Table 6-5, p. 227)

VI. Gastric motility disorders

A. Hirschprung disease (congenital aganglionic megacolon)

1. Description: congenital defect that results in mechanical obstruction from inadequate motility of an intestinal segment (Figure 6-1)

2. Etiology: may be accompanied by anomalies of other GI and genitourinary anomalies

3. Incidence
   a. Increased incidence in children with Down syndrome
   b. Follows a familial pattern of inheritance in some cases

4. Pathophysiology
   a. Absence of ganglion cells in an intestinal segment resulting in lack of peristalsis
   b. Bowel proximal to defect dilates because of a lack of peristalsis
   c. Failure of anal sphincter to relax; fecal matter accumulates in aganglionic segment

5. Assessment
   a. Assessment findings

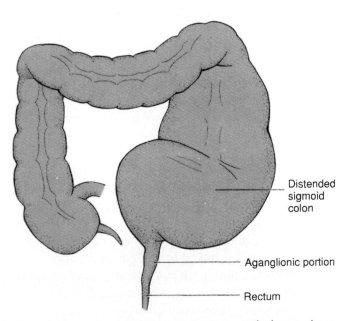

Figure 6-1. Hirschprung disease. (From Wong, D: *Whaley and Wong's nursing care of infants and children,* ed 5, St Louis, 1995, Mosby.)

(1) Neonatal period
  (a) Failure to pass meconium within 48 hours after birth
  (b) Bile-stained vomitus
  (c) Abdominal distention
(2) Early childhood
  (a) Ribbon-like stools
  (b) Constipation
  (c) Foul-smelling stools
  (d) Visible peristalsis
  (e) Recurrent diarrhea

b. Diagnostic procedures
  (1) Barium enema—reveals narrowed segment of bowel
  (2) Rectal biopsy—reveals absence of aganglion cells
  (3) Abdominal x-ray—reveals dilated loops of intestine
  (4) Rectal manometry—reveals failure of internal sphincter to relax

6. Therapeutic management
  a. Medications: preoperative antibiotics
  b. Treatments: enema therapy, nasogastric (NG) tube placement
  c. Surgery: two-stage process
    (1) Temporary colostomy construction
    (2) Resection of aganglionic segment; anastomosis of the intact ganglion segment to the rectum is performed during a "pull-through" procedure
  d. Colostomy closure usually occurs 3 months following the pull-through

7. Nursing management
  a. Acute care: preoperative
    (1) Nursing diagnoses
      (a) Altered nutrition: less than body requirements
      (b) Fluid volume deficit
    (2) Expected outcome: nutritional status is promoted before surgery, with fluid volume restored
    (3) Interventions
      (a) Assess child's weight, I&O, abdominal girth, fluid and electrolyte status
      (b) Offer diet high in calories and protein, low in residue
  b. Acute care: postoperative
    (1) Nursing diagnoses: same as preoperative

          (2) Expected outcome: nutritional status is maintained without dehydration or negative nitrogen balance

          (3) Interventions

              (a) Monitor child's hydration status including NG, colostomy, and indwelling urinary catheter drainage; IV, NG, and oral intake

              (b) Maintain patency of NG tube

              (c) Monitor return of bowel sounds, usually within 48 to 72 hours

    c. Home care

          (1) Nursing diagnosis: knowledge deficit

          (2) Expected outcome: parents demonstrate ability to provide enema therapy or ostomy care

          (3) Interventions

              (a) Provide instructions regarding colostomy care: the use and care of equipment, skin care, colostomy irrigation

              (b) Provide information regarding dietary management including high-residue or normal diet, adequate fluid intake

              (c) Encourage the verbalization of feelings related to the colostomy

    d. Additional nursing diagnoses

          (1) Constipation

          (2) Ineffective family coping

          (3) Impaired skin integrity

  8. Evaluation

    a. Parents provide colostomy care using proper technique

    b. Dehydration is prevented

    c. Nutritional status is restored

B. Gastroesophageal reflux (GER)

  1. Description: presence of stomach contents in the esophagus

  2. Etiology: exact cause unknown

  3. Incidence: predisposing factor is delayed maturation of esophageal neuromuscular control

  4. Pathophysiology

    a. Gastric-content reflux results in tissue inflammation and stricture—an abnormal temporary or permanent narrowing of a hollow organ

    b. Caused by incompetent cardiac sphincter at the esophageal–gastric junction

    c. The following effects occur as a result of GER
- (1) Esophagitis
- (2) Aspiration of gastric contents
- (3) Pulmonary disease
- (4) Esophageal stricture

    d. Complications of GER
- (1) Aspiration pneumonia
- (2) Apnea with cyanosis
- (3) Esophageal carcinoma

5. Assessment
    a. Assessment findings
- (1) Chronic vomiting
- (2) Failure to thrive
- (3) Esophageal bleeding manifested by hematemesis or melena

    b. Diagnostic procedures
- (1) Esophageal manometry—reveals lower esophageal sphincter pressure
- (2) Barium esophogram—reveals reflux
- (3) Intraesophageal pH monitoring—reveals pH of distal esophagus with reflux contents

6. Therapeutic management
    a. Medications
- (1) Cholinergics
   - (a) Bethanecol (Urecholine)—to increase esophageal tone and peristaltic activity; give before feeding
   - (b) Metoclopromide (Reglan)—to decrease esophageal pressure by relaxing pyloric and duodenal segments, increasing peristalsis without stimulating secretions
- (2) H_2 histamine receptor antagonists: cimetidine (Tagamet), Ranitidine HCl (Zantac)—to decrease gastric acidity and pepsin secretion; give before feeding
- (3) Antacids: to neutralize gastric acid between feedings; give after feeding (Maalox)

    b. Surgery: if reflux is severe, Nissen fundoplication is done—the creation of a valve mechanism by wrapping the greater curvature of the stomach (fundus) around the distal esophagus

7. Nursing management
    a. Acute care: preoperative

          (1) Nursing diagnosis: altered nutrition—less than body requirements

          (2) Expected outcome: child maintains or reestablishes adequate nutrient and fluid intake

          (3) Interventions

             (a) Assess feeding patterns, routines, and environment

             (b) Record vomitus: amount, characteristics, and frequency

             (c) Assess for signs of dehydration

             (d) Thicken formula with baby cereal (1 tsp/oz) to minimize reflux

             (e) Feed slowly; burp often (q 1 oz)

             (f) Handle child minimally after feedings

             (g) Position child as ordered; usually prone with head of mattress at 30 degree angle for infants >9 months of age; <9 months may use infant seat with infant supine

  b. Home care: postoperative

          (1) Nursing diagnosis: anxiety

          (2) Expected outcome: parental anxiety is reduced to a manageable level

          (3) Interventions

             (a) Assess family's concerns and available support systems

             (b) Provide opportunities for parents to express fears; identify coping strategies and education needs

             (c) Instruct parents about proper feeding techniques, positioning of child

             (d) Prepare parents for possibility of postsurgical problems such as gas bloat, choking on solids, and delayed gastric emptying

  c. Additional nursing diagnoses

          (1) Ineffective airway clearance

          (2) Fluid volume deficit

          (3) Knowledge deficit

          (4) Altered parenting

8. Evaluation

  a. Reflux activity minimized as family adheres to preventive measures

  b. Family exhibits decreased anxiety about illness and child care

  c. Family demonstrates proper technique for feeding and assessment techniques for complications

  d. Infant gains or maintains weight

VII. Obstructive disorders

A. Pyloric stenosis

1. Description: hypertrophy of circular muscle of the pylorus, causing narrowing of pyloric canal between the stomach and duodenum
2. Etiology: cause of pyloric muscle hypertrophy is unknown
3. Incidence
   a. Most commonly seen between 1 and 6 months of age
   b. Occurs mainly in full-term male infants as a congenital disorder; may also be acquired
4. Pathophysiology
   a. Narrowed pyloric canal gradually becomes obstructed; inflammation and edema result in a complete obstruction (Figure 6-2)
   b. Pyloric muscle enlarges to twice its usual size; stomach dilates
   c. Clinical picture develops gradually; in early stage of hypertrophy infant appears and eats well
   d. Vomiting progresses from mild regurgitation to projectile vomiting
5. Assessment
   a. Assessment findings
      (1) Vomiting: usually shortly after feeding; child will then appear hungry and accept more food
      (2) Emesis contains gastric contents, is nonbilous (no yellow-brown color), and is possibly blood tinged
      (3) Failure to gain weight or has a weight loss
      (4) Upper abdominal distention: palpable olive-shaped mass in epigastrium to right of umbilicus
      (5) Peristaltic waves visible from left to right across epigastrium
      (6) Signs of dehydration apparent as vomiting increases in frequency and amount
   b. Diagnostic procedures
      (1) Laboratory studies
         (a) Serum electrolytes: increased Na and K^+, decreased chloride
         (b) Arterial blood gases (ABGs) increased pH and bicarbonate indicating metabolic alkalosis from loss of hydrochloric stomach acid
         (c) Urine pH is increased
         (d) Increased Hgb and Hct result from extracellular fluid depletion; hemoconcentration

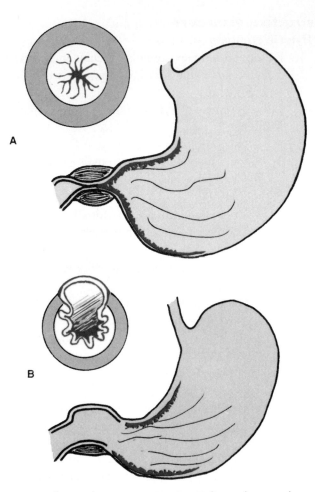

Figure 6-2. Hypertrophic pyloric stenosis. **A,** Enlarged muscular tumor nearly obliterates pyloric channel. **B,** Longitudinal surgical division of muscle down to submucosa establishes adequate passageway. (From Wong, D: *Whaley and Wong's nursing care of infants and children,* ed 5, St Louis, 1995, Mosby.)

       (2) Diagnostic procedures
          (a) Ultrasound reveals narrowing of the pyloric canal; preferred procedure, since less risk of aspiration of contrast medium
          (b) X-ray of upper abdomen with barium reveals delayed gastric emptying and elongation of the pyloric canal
    6. Therapeutic management
       a. Medications

        (1) Analgesics—for postoperative pain management

        (2) Antibiotics—to prevent postoperative infection

   b. Surgery: pyloromyotomy—incision through muscle fibers of pylorus: Fredet-Ramstedt procedure

7. Nursing management

   a. Acute care: preoperative

        (1) Nursing diagnosis: risk for fluid volume deficit

        (2) Expected outcomes

           (a) Fluid and electrolyte balance are maintained

           (b) Dehydration is prevented

           (c) Acid-base balance is maintained

        (3) Interventions

           (a) Asses frequency and volume of vomiting after feedings

           (b) Assess hydration status: daily weights, I&O, urine specific gravity

           (c) Monitor for signs of dehydration

           (d) Monitor serum electrolytes and ABGs

           (e) Administer IV fluids as ordered

           (f) Maintain patency of gastric tube (if present)

   b. Postoperative/home care

        (1) Nursing diagnoses

           (a) Knowledge deficit

           (b) Altered nutrition: less than body requirements

        (2) Expected outcomes

           (a) Adequate nutrition is maintained

           (b) Parents verbalize correct feeding technique and follow-up care

        (3) Interventions

           (a) Begin small, frequent feedings postoperatively: begin with glucose water, advance to dilute, then full-strength formula

           (b) Feed in upright position, burp frequently

           (c) Handle minimally after feedings

           (d) Position on right side, with head elevated, after feedings

           (e) Assess family's knowledge of the disease and readiness to learn

           (f) Demonstrate feeding procedure and incision care

           (g) Provide opportunities for parents to assume infant's care before discharge

      c. Additional nursing diagnoses
          (1) Risk for injury
          (2) Anxiety
          (3) Alteration in comfort
  8. Evaluation
      a. Child maintains weight, acid-base and fluid balance
      b. Parents appropriately care for child, feed, and care for incision before hospital discharge

B. Intussusception
  1. Description: telescoping of one portion of bowel into another portion, resulting in obstruction to passage of intestinal contents (Figure 6-3)
  2. Etiology: cause unknown
  3. Incidence
      a. Most common cause of intestinal obstruction in the first 2 years of life
      b. Children at risk are those diagnosed with cystic fibrosis, celiac disease, and gastroenteritis

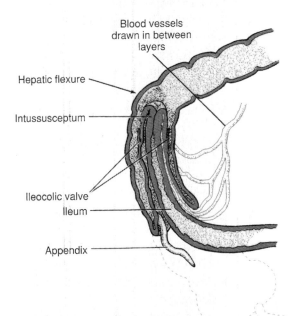

Figure 6-3. Ileocolic intussusception. (From Wong, D: *Whaley and Wong's nursing care of infants and children*, ed 5, St Louis, 1995, Mosby.)

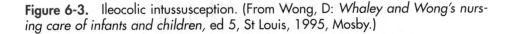

4. Pathophysiology
   a. Inflammation and ischemia occur in the intestinal wall as portions press against each other
   b. Eventual tissue necrosis, perforation, and peritonitis may occur
5. Assessment
   a. Assessment findings
      (1) Paroxysmal, acute pain in abdomen
      (2) Vomiting
      (3) "Currant-jellylike" stools
      (4) Cylindrical mass above affected area
   b. Diagnostic procedures—abdominal x-ray and barium enema—reveal affected area of intestine
6. Therapeutic management
   a. Treatment: hydrostatic reduction by barium enema
   b. Surgery: performed if reduction by barium enema is not successful or tissue necrosis is present
   c. Medications
      (1) Antibiotics to treat peritonitis
      (2) Analgesics to manage postoperative pain
7. Nursing management
   a. Acute care
      (1) Nursing diagnoses
         (a) Risk for injury
         (b) Knowledge deficit
      (2) Expected outcome: child's bowel pattern returns to normal
      (3) Interventions
         (a) Assess child for findings of intussusception
         (b) Maintain patency of NG tube; size appropriate for age
         (c) Administer IV fluids as ordered
         (d) Inform parents of rationale for NG tube and NPO status; NG tube size depends on child's size, weight, and fluid to be infused

Age	Catheter size (FR)
newborns and infants	5 to 6, 8
>6 yr	8 to 10
adolescent	12 to 16

         (e) Inform parents of possible need for surgery if barium enema does not reduce invagination

      b. Postoperative care

          (1) Nursing diagnosis: risk for fluid volume deficit

          (2) Expected outcomes

               (a) Child maintains or regains hydration status

               (b) Child tolerates daily intake of fluid requirements

          (3) Interventions

               (a) Assess fluid intake and output every 8 hours

               (b) Weigh child daily

               (c) Maintain intravenous therapy as ordered

               (d) Monitor child for signs of dehydration

               (e) Reestablish fluid feedings; offer clear fluids and progress slowly to solids

          (4) Nursing diagnosis: alteration in bowel elimination

          (5) Expected outcome: child demonstrates normal bowel pattern

          (6) Interventions

               (a) Assess child for return of bowel sounds

               (b) Monitor child for passage of stool and or barium (barium stool will be whitish-clay–colored)

               (c) Inform parents that elimination of brown stools indicates that invagination has been corrected

    8. Evaluation

      a. Family verbalizes information regarding therapies, procedures, findings to report to physician

      b. Child displays absence of complications or recurrence of invagination of bowel

VIII. Malabsorption: celiac disease (gluten enteropathy)

    A. Description: intolerance to gluten, the protein component of wheat, barley, rye, and oats; causes impairment of absorptive processes

    B. Etiology: symptoms of disorder occur 3 to 6 months following introduction of gluten-containing grains into diet; usually before 2 years of age

    C. Incidence

        1. Evidence supports genetic link in occurrence of disorder

        2. Mainly found in the Caucasian population

    D. Pathophysiology

        1. Gliadin fraction of gluten causes damage to mucosal cells; villi atrophy, causing malabsorption (Figure 6-4)

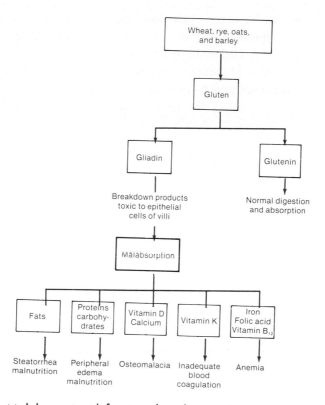

Figure 6-4. Malabsorptive defect in celiac disease. (From Wong, D: *Whaley and Wong's nursing care of infants and children,* ed 5, St Louis, 1995, Mosby.)

    2. Initially, fat absorption is impaired; later, protein and carbohydrate absorption are also impaired

    3. Cystic fibrosis has many of the clinical features that are also seen in celiac disease (Table 6-6, p. 228)

E. Assessment

    1. Assessment findings

        a. Early signs

            (1) Diarrhea; failure to regain weight following diarrheal episode

            (2) Constipation

            (3) Vomiting

            (4) Abdominal pain

            (5) Steatorrhea—fatty stools

        b. Later signs

            (1) Behavioral changes: irritability, apathy

            (2) Muscle wasting, with loss of subcutaneous fat

      c. Celiac crisis—rare event that requires immediate medical intervention

         (1) Severe dehydration

         (2) Metabolic acidosis

  2. Diagnostic procedures

      (1) Laboratory studies: stool analysis—reveals steatorrhea

      (2) Diagnostic studies

         (a) Jejunal biopsy—reveals atrophy of mucosal cells

         (b) Serum antigliadin and antireticulin antibodies—presence indicative of disorder

         (c) Sweat test—to rule out cystic fibrosis

F. Therapeutic management

  1. Medications

      a. Vitamin supplements: fat-soluble supplements (A, D, E, K) supplied in water-miscible form

      b. Mineral supplements

      c. Steroids—used in celiac crisis to decrease bowel inflammation

  2. Treatments: dietary management

      a. Gluten-free diet: substitute corn, rice, or millet as grain source

      b. Lifelong elimination of gluten sources: wheat, rye, oats and barley

G. Nursing management

  1. Acute care

      a. Nursing diagnoses

         (1) Altered nutrition: less than body requirements

         (2) Knowledge deficit

      b. Expected outcomes

         (1) Child adheres to prescribed diet

         (2) Child's growth and development are adequate

      c. Interventions

         (1) Assess for findings of celiac disease

         (2) Discuss parental concerns about the diagnosis and implications of the treatment regimen

         (3) Instruct parents on gluten-free diet: the elimination of oats, wheat, barley, and rye substances throughout life

         (4) Teach parents methods to prevent celiac crisis: adherence to diet, prevention of stress and infection

  2. Home care

      a. Nursing diagnosis: anxiety

        b. Expected outcomes
           (1) Family integrates disease prevention into lifestyle
           (2) Family expresses reduced anxiety
        c. Interventions
           (1) Provide parents opportunities for expression of fears and concerns related to the disease and its impact on their lifestyle
           (2) Provide support group information to the family; refer if indicated
           (3) Discuss alternate ways to cope with fears and anxieties
    3. Additional nursing diagnoses
        a. Risk for fluid volume deficit
        b. Diarrhea
        c. Noncompliance
  H. Evaluation
    1. Family identifies acceptable and unacceptable foods in diet
    2. Child maintains symptom-free state
    3. Parents exhibit less anxiety and effective coping resources

IX. Inflammatory disorder: appendicitis

  A. **Description: inflammation of appendix, a blind sac connected to end of cecum; may lead to perforation, peritonitis, and sepsis if left untreated**
  B. **Etiology**
    1. Caused by obstruction of the lumen of the appendix; most commonly a result of a fecalith or hardened feces
    2. Other causes are lymphoid hyperplasia, tumors, fibrotic stenosis; other factors possibly implicated are worms and a low-fiber diet
  C. **Incidence**
    1. Rapid progression to peritonitis is characteristic in infants and young children
    2. Occurs mainly in school-age children and adolescents
  D. **Pathophysiology**
    1. Lumen obstruction causes blocking of mucous secretion; blood vessels become compressed; ischemia results
    2. Bacterial invasion and necrosis subsequently occur
    3. Acute inflammation rapidly progresses to perforation and peritonitis if left undiagnosed

E. **Assessment**
1. Assessment findings
   a. Appendicitis
      (1) Pain, cramping initially located in periumbilical area; descends to right lower quadrant; most intense at McBurney's point—located midway between the anterior superior iliac crest and the umbilicus; occasionally pain is severe suprapubic
      (2) Rebound tenderness and abdominal rigidity
      (3) Low-grade fever <100° F orally
      (4) Vomiting, nausea
      (5) Constipation or diarrhea
      (6) Side-lying position with abdominal guarding; legs flexed
   b. Peritonitis
      (1) Fever increases
      (2) Progressive abdominal distention
      (3) Increase in abdominal pain
      (4) Rigid guarding of abdomen
      (5) Tachycardia; tachypnea
      (6) Pallor, chills, and restlessness
2. Diagnostic procedures
   a. Laboratory studies
      (1) CBC: WBC count increases to 15,000-20,000, usually with polymorphonuclear leukocytosis
      (2) Urinalysis—reveals pyuria
   b. Diagnostic studies
      (1) Abdominal x-ray—reveals presence of fecalith in appendix
      (2) Ultrasound—reveals location of abscess before surgery
F. **Therapeutic management**
1. Surgery: appendectomy—surgical removal of appendix before perforation
2. Medications
   a. Analgesics—narcotic and nonnarcotic for control of postoperative pain
   b. Antibiotics—systemic; usually only given if rupture or abscess to treat peritonitis
3. Treatments following rupture of appendix
   a. Preoperative IV fluids, IV antibiotics, NG suction

   b. Postoperative: external drainage such as penrose drains;
       wound irrigations, since incision may be left open to heal
       from inside out
G. **Nursing management**
   1. Acute care: preoperative
       a. Nursing diagnosis: alteration in comfort
       b. Expected outcome: pain is reduced or eliminated
       c. Interventions
           (1) Assess pain: location, severity, character; check for
                rebound tenderness
           (2) Assess vital signs, noting tachycardia, shallow, fast
                respirations and fever >100° F
           (3) Keep NPO
           (4) Provide comfort measures: analgesics; frequent
                mouth care antipyretics will be minimally effective if
                appendix is abscessed; right side-lying or low- to
                semifowler's position to promote comfort or to
                localize abscess when appendix ruptures
           (5) Apply ice packs to abdomen for 20 to 30 min q 1 hr;
                avoid application of heat
           (6) Report any changes in type, level, or location of
                pain; typically if appendix ruptures, pain stops or
                significantly decreases
           (7) Provide diversional activity for quiet play
           (8) Avoid use of laxatives or enemas
   2. Postoperative
       a. Nursing diagnoses
           (1) Risk for infection
           (2) Knowledge deficit
       b. Expected outcome: child's incision remains free of
           infection
       c. Interventions
           (1) Assess incision for signs of infection: redness,
                swelling, pain, character of drainage
           (2) Assess incision for presence of penrose drain; if
                present, drainage may be profuse for the initial 12
                hours; maintain NG suction and patency which is
                usually present if rupture occurred
           (3) Position in right side-lying or low- to semifowler's
                position with legs flexed to facilitate drainage
           (4) Change dressing as ordered or reinforce as
                necessary; record type and amount of drainage

             (5)   Administer antibiotics and analgesics as ordered

             (6)   If an open incision, teach parents sterile wound care, irrigation, and packing technique. May use wet or dry dressings

             (7)   Monitor temperature for elevations

    3. Additional nursing diagnoses

        a. Anxiety

        b. Risk for fluid volume deficit

        c. Diarrhea/constipation

        d. Hyperthermia

        e. Altered nutrition: less than body requirements

H. Evaluation

    1. Incision heals without infection

    2. Preoperative and postoperative pain relieved or controlled with ordered medications

    3. If open incision, parents perform sterile technique for process of irrigating, packing, and dressing wound

    4. Parents state findings to report to the physician

Table 6-1. Summary of Major Gastrointestinal Diagnostic Procedures

Procedure	Function	Indications	Nursing Considerations
Stool Examination			
Ova and parasites	Examination of stool for presence of organisms	Parasite infestation	Requires fresh, warm specimen
Fat	Aids in diagnosis of pancreatic insufficiency	Cystic fibrosis Celiac disease Malabsorption syndrome	Child's stool needs to be collected for 72 hours in one container. No special preservatives used.
Occult blood, guiac	Detects presence of blood in stool	Infection Inflammation Ulcerative colitis	Requires stool collection usually × 3, each specimen sent to lab individually
Endoscopy			
Upper GI-esophagogas-troduodenoscopy	Use of fiberoptic endoscope Allows visualization of mucosal lining of esophagus, stomach, and duodenum	Foreign body removal Inflammatory disorders Vomiting of blood	Young child must be restrained; procedure may have to be done under general anesthesia Position during procedure is left lateral decubitus Withhold fluids until child is alert and swallow (gag) reflex returns, usually 2 to 4 hours

Modified from Wong, D: *Whaley and Wong's nursing care of infants and children*, ed 5, St Louis, 1995, Mosby.

217

Table 6-2. Commonly Used Gastrointestinal Medication for Children

Classification	Medication	Indications	Route and Dosage	Side Effects	Nursing Implications
Antibiotic, sulfonamide Functional classification: antiinflam-matory	Generic: sulfa-salazine Trade: Azulfidine	Inflammatory bowel disease—Chron's disease	PO >2 years Loading dose: 40-60 mg/kg/day in 3 to 6 equally divided doses Maintenance dose: 30 mg/kg/day in 4 equally divided doses	*CNS:* Headache, lethargy *GI:* Nausea, vomiting, diarrhea *GU:* Crystalluria, hematuria, orange-yellow color to alkaline urine *Integumentary:* Orange-yellow color to skin, urticaria, rash, photosensitivity	Assess previous allergies to sulfanamides, antibiotics Administer total daily dose in evenly spaced doses and after meals to help minimize GI intolerance Shake suspension well; may crush tablet and give with small amount of food Observe for hypersensitivity Monitor CBC for decreased H+H, WBC Monitor UA for crystalluria during treatment Encourage PO fluid intake of at least 2000 cc/day to prevent crystalluria

Antibiotic, sulfonomide —cont'd					*Parent education:* Administer full course of therapy Protect child from sun; sunscreens may be ineffective Administer each dose with at least 6 ounces of water
Broad-spectrum antibiotic, penicillin	Generic: ampicillin Trade: Omnipen	Appendicitis; peritonitis	PO child >1 month 50-100 mg/kg/day in divided doses q 6 to 8 hr IV 50-100 mg/kg/day in divided doses q 6 to 12 hr	*CNS:* Lethargy, convulsions *GI:* Nausea, vomiting, diarrhea *GU:* Vaginitis, moniliasis *Integumentary:* Pruritic rash *Hematology:* Anemia, thrombo-cytopenia *Other:* Anaphylaxis	Assess previous allergy to penicillin and cephalosporins Assess for symptoms of yeast infections in females Administer oral ampicillin on empty stomach with glass of water to facilitate absorption: 1 to 2 hours AC or 2 to 3 hours PC Monitor liver studies Observe for allergic reaction by taking vital signs, especially respiratory effort, and checking skin for rash (usually on abdomen or upper torso)

Continued.

Table 6-2. Commonly Used Gastrointestinal Medication for Children—cont'd

Classification	Medication	Indications	Route and Dosage	Side Effects	Nursing Implications
Broad spectrum antibiotic —cont'd					Administer IV or IM solution within 1 hr of preparation Refrigerate oral suspension, shake well before use, and use within 2 weeks *Parent education:* Child should complete entire course of treatment Report diarrhea or rash to physician
Antacid	Generic: aluminum hydroxide Trade: Mylanta, Alternagel Basaljel	Gastritis Peptic ulcers Gastroesophageal reflux	PO *Ulcer therapy:* 5-15 ml/dose q 3 to 6 hr *GI bleeding therapy:* Infants: 2-15 ml/dose q 1 to 2 hr Children: 5-15 ml/dose q 1 to 2 hr	*GI:* Constipation anorexia, intestinal obstruction, fecal impaction *Other:* Dementia (aluminum toxicity)	Shake well before administration Assess for constipation Maintain fluid intake for age *Parent education:* Avoid OTC medication unless physician is consulted Monitor for constipation

Classification	Generic/Trade	Use	Dosage	Side effects	Nursing considerations
Antacid	Generic: magaldrate (hydroxymagnesium aluminate) Trade: Riopan	Peptic ulcer Gastroesophageal reflux Hiatal hernia	PO Peptic ulcer: 5-15 ml/dose q 3 to 6 hr Other conditions: dosage variable; depends on indication	*GI:* Constipation, diarrhea *Other:* Hypermagnesemia, especially in presence of impaired renal function	Shake well before administration Give with small amount of H_2O Assess stool consistency and pattern Maintain fluid intake *Parent education:* Administer according to prescribed dosage Do not give with other OTC medications without physician consultation
Anticholinergic	Generic: propantheline Trade: Pro-banthine	Control diarrhea associated with inflammatory bowel disease by decreasing peristalsis	PO Child: 1.5 mg/kg/day in 4 divided doses	*CNS:* Dizziness, headache, insomnia *CV:* Palpitations tachycardia *GI:* Dry mouth, paralytic ileus *GU:* Urinary retention *Integumentary:* Urticaria, pruritis *Sensory:* Blurred vision *Other:* Anaphylaxis	Obtain baseline vital signs *Parent education:* Monitor CNS symptoms for indication of overdosage—mainly decreased LOC Crush tablet and mix with small amount of food or fluid Sugarless gum or candy will relieve dry mouth Drug may cause blurred vision

Continued.

221

Table 6-2. Commonly Used Gastrointestinal Medication for Children—cont'd

Classification	Medication	Indications	Route and Dosage	Side Effects	Nursing Implications
Anticholinergic	Generic: glyco-pyrrolate Trade: Robinul	Peptic ulcer Other GI diseases associated with hyper-motility, hyperacidity, and spasm	PO >12 years: 1 mg TID IM/IV 0.1-0.2 mg as single dose Contraindicated in children <3 years of age	*CNS:* Drowsiness, weakness, headache *CV:* Palpitations, tachycardia *GI:* Constipation *GU:* Urinary hesitancy *EENT:* Blurred vision, photophobia *Integumentary:* Rash	Monitor vital signs Monitor I&O *Parent education:* Avoid high environmental temperature Monitor for rash, blurred vision Advise use of sunglasses
H₂ histamine receptor antagonist	Generic: cimetidine Trade: Tagamet	Gastro-esophageal reflux Peptic ulcer disease	PO 20-40 mg/kg/day in doses QID IM, IV 20-40 mg/kg/day in equally divided doses q 6 hr (maximum dose 2400 mg/day)	*CNS:* Dizziness, headache *CV:* Bradycardia *GI:* Diarrhea *GU:* Increased BUN *Hematology:* Neutropenia *Integumentary:* Rash, dermatitis *Other:* Muscular pain	Monitor blood counts, renal and hepatic function during treatment Assess mental and neurologic status *Parent education:* Administer 30 minutes before or with meals Tablet may be crushed Do not stop medication or take OTC medications without physician consultation

H₂ histamine receptor antagonist	Generic: ranitidine hydrochloride Trade: Zantac	Peptic ulcer GE reflux	PO 2-4 mg/kg/day in doses q 12 hr IM, IV 1-2 mg/kg/day in equally divided doses q 6-8 hrs	*CNS:* Dizziness, malaise *CV:* Bradycardia *GI:* Nausea, constipation *Skin:* Rash, urticaria	*Parent education:* May administer 30 minutes before or with meals Tablets may be crushed and mixed with food Notify physician if side effects occur Child should not take OTC medication without consulting physician

Table 6-3. Overview of Types of Dehydration

Dehydration Type	Pathology	Assessment Findings
Isotonic	Proportionate loss of water and electrolytes Occur with large amount of liquid stools, vomiting, hemorrhage, burns, fever	Thirst Acute weight loss Dry skin and mucous membranes Sunken eyeballs Lethargy Cold extremities Oliguria Hypovolemia
Hypertonic (hypernatremia)	Water lost in excess of electrolytes Osmotic gradient between ECF and ICF causes water to move out of cells into ECF Occurs with gastroenteritis in infants fed high-solute replacement fluids Seen in children with fever accompanied by hyperventilation May be seen with diabetes mellitus	Altered CNS status —lethargy Decreased urine output and skin turgor Weight loss Thirst Muscle rigidity
Hypotonic	Electrolytes lost in excess of water Osmotic gradient between ECF and ICF causes water movement into cell Accompanies diarrhea syndrome for inappropriate antidiuretic hormone	Irritability, seizures, coma Dry mucous membranes Decreased urine output Rapid, thready pulse Weight loss Shock

Table 6-4. Common Causes of Acute Pediatric Gastroenteritis

Organism/ Disease Factor/ Treatment	Age Affected	Assessment Findings	Pathology	Transmission	Peak Incidence
Viral Agents					
Rotavirus Prevent dehydration	6 to 24 months	Fever Vomiting Diarrhea	Mucosal atrophy Inflammation	Person-to-person	Winter
Norwalk virus Prevent dehydration	All	Fever Anorexia Vomiting	Inflammation of mucosa Villi damage	Person-to-person	Winter
Bacterial agents					
Escherichia coli (E. coli) Antibiotics Prevent dehydration Antispasmodics	0 to 18 months	Green liquid stools Fever Vomiting	Enterotoxin production Invasion of GI epithelium	Person-to-person Ingestion of contaminated food, water, inanimate objects	All year, especially summer
Salmonella No specific treatment Major goal: prevent dehydration Antibiotics typically not indicated	0 to 2 years	6 to 48 hr after eating contaminated food a sudden onset of diarrhea, watery stools contain blood, pus, or mucus Colicky abdominal pain Vomiting Fever	Invasion of GI mucosa Symptoms may last 2 to 5 days	Contaminated food and drink from animal sources—eggs, poultry, milk	Year-round, especially July through October

Continued.

Table 6-4. Common Causes of Acute Pediatric Gastroenteritis—cont'd

Organism/ Disease Factor/ Treatment	Age Affected	Assessment Findings	Pathology	Transmission	Peak Incidence
Shigella Preferred treatment: supportive Likelihood of encountering antibiotic - resistant organisms is high Major goal: prevent dehydration	0 to 10 years	Diarrhea, stools contain pus Fever Abdominal pain Tenesmus— persistent, ineffective spasms of rectum accompanied by a desire to empty bowel; may be painful	Enterotoxin production	Person-to-person Isolation and strict handwashing precautions essential	Late summer Must be reported to public health department
Food poisoning					
Staphylococcal Prevent dehydration Bed rest Analgesics Antimicrobials that are resistant to penicillinase	All	Nausea Vomiting Severe abdominal cramping Occurs 6 to 12 hours after ingestion of contaminated food	Enterotoxin production	Contaminated food sources —inadequately cooled or refrigerated (e.g., custards, mayonnaise)	Year-round

Modified from Wong, D: *Whaley and Wong's nursing care of infants and children*, ed 5, St Louis, 1995, Mosby.

Table 6-5. Common Accidental Ingestions

Ingestion	Assessment Findings	Treatment	Priority Nursing Interventions
Acetaminophen (Tylenol)	Nausea, vomiting Pallor Liver involvement—jaundice, stupor, coagulation abnormalities	Induce emesis Mucomyst, PO, usually QID × 3-4 days Activated charcoal	Monitor tests for liver function —ALT, AST Teach parents proper administration and dosage of acetaminophen

Salicylate (aspirin)	Tinnitus
	Hyperventilation
	Initially:
	  Respiratory alkalosis
	  Metabolic acidosis
		Induce emesis or gastric lavage
		IV fluids and electrolytes
		IV sodium bicarbonate if pH <7.2
		Vitamin K if bleeding
			Assess for bleeding
			Monitor renal function—serum creatinine
			Caution parents to avoid giving aspirin to children to prevent Reye's syndrome

Hydrocarbons (e.g., gasoline, kerosene)	Nausea, vomiting Altered sensorium Weakness Pulmonary involvement— cyanosis, tachypnea, sternal retractions	Administer O$_2$ Treatment controversial; depends on agent ingested	Remove clothing and wash skin in contact with poison Monitor vital signs Support ventilation Support parents
Corrosives (e.g., strong acids or alkalis as found in household cleaning products and drain cleaner)	Mouth, throat, and stomach burning Edema of lips, tongue, and pharynx Drooling Signs of shock Anxiety Vomiting, hemoptysis	Vomiting contraindicated Dilute agents with water Analgesics for pain NPO May insert gastric tube	Ensure patent airway Monitor vital signs, LOC Monitor acid-base status Support parents

Table 6-6 Comparison of Celiac Disease and Cystic Fibrosis

Metabolic Disorder	Age of Onset	Etiology	Assessment Findings	Diagnostic Tests	Treatment
Celiac disease	9 to 12 months	Unknown	Diarrhea—pale, foul smelling Anemia Growth retardation Muscle wasting	Biopsy of bowel Sweat test	High-protein, high-calorie, gluten-free diet—avoid pasta and breads made with barley, oats, rye, wheat Vitamins A, D, E, K, in water-soluble form Use foods made from rice, corn, or millet
Cystic fibrosis	0 to 6 months	Autosomal recessive disorder	Newborn: Meconium ileus Steatorrhea from impaired fat digestion Chronic hypoxia, respiratory infections Increased sweat electrolytes (Na, Cl) Increased viscosity of bronchial mucus	Sweat test	*Pulmonary:* Chest physiotherapy Antibiotic and aerosol therapy *GI:* Pancreatic enzymes given with meals High-protein, high-calorie, and low-fat diet Give vitamins A, D, E, K, in water-soluble forms

REVIEW QUESTIONS

1. A preschooler has been recently diagnosed with celiac disease. Which of the following menu choices selected by the parents would indicate that effective instruction has occurred?
   a. Corn tortilla and fresh fruit salad
   b. Pizza and chocolate brownie
   c. Spaghetti and slice of pie
   d. Sandwich with bologna and ice cream

2. An infant is experiencing uncontrolled vomiting. Based on this finding, the nurse would expect which acid-base imbalance?
   a. Metabolic alkalosis
   b. Metabolic acidosis
   c. Respiratory alkalosis
   d. Respiratory acidosis

3. An infant has undergone surgical repair of bilateral cleft lip. Which of these goals should receive priority in the infant's immediate care?
   a. Adequate nutritional intake will be provided
   b. Family will be supported
   c. Trauma to suture line will be prevented
   d. Operative site will remain free of infection

4. A 4-week-old infant with a history of vomiting after feeding has been hospitalized with a tentative diagnosis of pyloric stenosis. Which of these actions should the nurse initially take?
   a. Begin an intravenous infusion
   b. Measure abdominal circumference
   c. Orient family member to unit
   d. Weigh infant

5. Following a pyloromyotomy, the nurse caring for an infant should expect to position the infant in which of the following ways?
   a. On the right side in a low fowler's position all the time
   b. In a prone position on a pillow only at night
   c. Slightly on the right side in an infant car seat after feeding
   d. Slightly on the left side with the head of the bed elevated after feeding

6. An infant is admitted to the hospital with a sudden episode of acute abdominal pain. To help establish a diagnosis of intussusception, the nurse should ask which question?
   a. "Did the infant have a recent infection?"
   b. "Has the infant had projectile vomiting?"
   c. "Does the infant's stool look like currant jelly?"
   d. "Do you burp the infant frequently while feeding?"

7. A toddler is admitted to the hospital with acute gastroenteritis. An intravenous infusion has been ordered. Before adding potassium to the IV solution, which of these actions should the nurse take?
   a. Check order with the physician
   b. Determine whether the child voided
   c. Monitor capillary refill
   d. Weigh the child

8. A parent receives preoperative instructions for an infant who is diagnosed with pyloric stenosis. Which of these statements by the mother indicates that she understands the instructions?
   a. "Feeding with formula may begin 6 hours after surgery"
   b. "Feeding with glucose water may begin 6 hours after surgery"
   c. "The baby cannot feed during the first 24 hours after surgery"
   d. "The baby will be started on formula immediately after surgery"

9. A staff member includes all of the following measures in caring for an infant who has had cleft lip repair surgery. Which of these actions indicates that the staff member needs additional coaching?
   a. Infant is placed in elbow restraints
   b. Infant is placed in prone position to facilitate drainage of secretions
   c. Infant's suture line is gently cleansed after feedings as ordered
   d. Restraints are removed periodically

10. Following instructions regarding a celiac crisis, which comment would indicate an understanding by the parents of these instructions?
    a. "Celiac crisis is not a serious complication"
    b. "My child must avoid exposure to infection"
    c. "Antihistamines are recommended"
    d. "Skipping a meal such as breakfast is not a problem"

ANSWERS, RATIONALES, AND TEST-TAKING TIPS

Rationales	Test-Taking Tips

1. **Correct answer: a**

    Celiac disease is characterized by an intolerance for a gliadin faction of gluten, a protein found in wheat, barley, rye, and oats. Corn, rice, and millet are substitute grains. All of the foods in options *b*, *c*, and *d* except the ice cream contain some degree of wheat, barley, rye, or oats.

    Remember the little story of B.O. from R.W. and stay away from both.
    B = *barley*
    O = *oats*
    R = *rye not rice*
    W = *wheat*

2. **Correct answer: a**

    Prolonged vomiting causes decreased chloride levels from the loss of hydrochloric acid from the stomach. The result is increased pH and bicarbonate, which are characteristic of metabolic alkalosis. Metabolic acidosis results from diarrhea, acute renal failure, diabetic ketoacidosis, and any massive trauma or insult to the body such as severe burns. Respiratory alkalosis is caused by an increase in the rate and depth of pulmonary ventilation with exhalation of large amounts of CO_2 where levels are <35 mm Hg on the blood gases. Respiratory acidosis results from diminished or inadequate pulmonary ventilation with an increased PCO_2 of >45 mm Hg in the blood gases.

    The first step is to remember that if the respiratory system is not involved, the problem is metabolic; thus, the correct response is either *a* or *b*. An easy way to remember metabolic imbalances with the gastrointestinal (GI) system is "loss of acid from the gut (stomach)," get a "body full of base" (metabolic alkalosis). In losses from the other end of the GI, the rectum, the opposite happens: "loss of base from the butt," get metabolic acidosis. One last tip: The body typically goes into a metabolic acidosis if any malfunction occurs, since tissues are better oxygenated in an acidotic state.

3. **Correct answer: c**

The major priority in the immediate postoperative period is the protection of the operative site to ensure optimum healing and cosmetic repair. Feeding is carried out in the same manner as before surgery. Physiological needs take priority in the immediate postoperative period. Option *d* is an appropriate goal in the postoperative period for the child needing cleft lip repair; however, protection from trauma is an immediate concern and the priority.

The time factor of "immediate" care postoperative is crucial. Otherwise, response *d* may have been selected istead of *c*, which is the correct answer. Response *d* would be correct if the question had asked about home care and education.

4. **Correct answer: d**

Weight provides the best assessment of the hydration status, which is a priority for an infant with a history of vomiting. Since emphasis of care involves restoring hydration and electrolyte balance, an IV infusion will be started following assessment of the hydration status. Option *b* is not an action associated with the care of a child with pyloric stenosis; it is an appropriate action for a client with abdominal ascites. Option *c* is not a priority action, yet it is appropriate once family members' anxiety is reduced and questions are answered.

Any client with the potential for fluid loss or gain is best evaluated for hydration by weight, usually done initially on admission and daily.

5. **Correct answer: c**

Infant is positioned in this manner to facilitate gastric emptying. Semi- to high fowler's position is preferred after feeding (not constantly) to decrease the possibility of vomiting and facilitate gastric emptying. Option *b* may be a position for an infant with gastroesophageal reflux. The position in option *d* hinders gastric emptying.

After reading the question and responses, take time to recall normal anatomy and physiology of the upper GI tract. The pyloric valve, which divides the stomach from the duodenum, is located in the upper right quadrant of the abdomen. Therefore, to facilitate gastric emptying, select the response in which the infant is turned to the right side and somewhat upright; gravity will help move the food downward.

6. **Correct answer: c**

As intussusception progresses, the affected infant demonstrates increased vomiting, apathy, and passage of stools mixed with blood and mucus, which looks like currant jelly. An antecedent infection is not part of the disease process. Projectile vomiting is a classic finding in pyloric stenosis. The disease process is not linked to feeding technique but is a structural abnormality of the intestine, the lower gastrointestinal tract. Feeding difficulties tend to be associated with upper gastrointestinal findings.

One approach is to eliminate responses *a, b,* and *d* as incorrect from your basic knowledge of GI diagnoses and findings. Also, note the key time frame "sudden acute." Options *a* and *d* would not indicate an acute problem. Projectile vomiting may lessen any pain, since it would result in less pressure in the GI tract.

7. **Correct answer: b**

If the child has voided, it establishes that adequate renal function is present.

Reread the responses and summarize each in this manner to clarify the information.

The actions in options *a* and *c* are not necessary before adding potassium to an IV fluid. A child with a history of acute gastroenteritis should be weighed at admission and on a daily basis. Weight would not influence a decision about potassium administration.

Response *a:* communication with physician
Response *b:* renal function
Response *c:* arterial circulation
Response *d:* hydration status
The priority data to associate with potassium administration would be renal function—response *b.*

8. Correct answer: b

Apply general concepts of providing oral fluids after any surgery: clear liquids to full liquids to solids, progressing according to tolerance of the client. In this client, postoperative feedings are usually instituted relatively soon, beginning with clear liquids that contain glucose and electrolytes such as Pediolyte. Formulas are considered full liquids. Feedings are instituted within the first 24 hours, unless contraindicated for some special reason.

The best approach to this question is to first look for a clear liquid substance—only found in response *b.* You may think response *c* is correct if you recall that for the postoperative GI tract, oral fluids are given only when bowel sounds return, usually after 48 to 72 hours in the adult. Now reread response *c;* it states "cannot feed . . . the first 24 hours." This statement is absolute and restrictive as written and therefore is probably not the correct response. Select response *b.*

9. Correct answer: b

Infants who have had cleft lip repair must be prevented from lying on their abdomens, which facilitates rubbing their faces on the sheets. In options *a, c,* and *d* the actions are correct with no need for further instruction. The use of elbow restraints is recommended to prevent infants from rubbing their

The process to select the correct answer is to make sure the question is reread after initially reading through the responses. This helps to clarify that an incorrect action must be selected.

incisions. Cleansing after feedings prevents infection and enhances healing. The suture line is cleansed of formula as needed. Removal of the restraints one at a time with supervision allows for exercise of the arms and allows for stimulation and body contact.

10. **Correct answer: b**

Exacerbation of celiac disease—crisis—can be prevented by adhering to a gluten-free diet and preventing the child's contact with individuals who have an infection. Celiac crisis, although rare, is a serious complication that requires prompt medical intervention to correct dehydration and metabolic acidosis. Drugs with anticholinergic effects such as antihistamines, which may precipitate a celiac crisis, must be avoided. Meals should be eaten on a regular basis.

If you have no idea of the correct response, select the response that pertains to infection rather than the other responses.

▼ ▼ ▼ ▼ ▼ ▼ ▼ ▼ ▼ ▼ ▼ ▼ ▼ ▼

Nursing Care of Children with Genitourinary and Renal Disorders

STUDY OUTCOMES

After completing this chapter, the reader will be able to do the following:

▼ Discuss the kidney's role in maintaining fluid and electrolyte balance.

▼ List common blood and urine tests to determine renal function.

▼ Identify nursing diagnoses that are commonly applied to the child with altered renal function.

▼ Outline a plan of care for a child with vesicoureteral reflux.

▼ Compare assessment findings and nursing care of a child with nephrotic syndrome and a child with acute glomerulonephritis.

▼ Outline nursing care typically needed for the family of a child who has a structural defect of the genitourinary system.

KEY TERMS

Albumin	Water-soluble, heat-coagulable protein; can be given IV as a plasma-volume expander.
Ambiguous genitalia	External genitalia that are not normal and morphologically typical of either sex, as occurs in pseudohermaphroditism.
Dysuria	Painful urination, usually the result of a bacterial infection or obstructive condition in the urinary tract.
Erythropoietin	Glycoprotein hormone synthesized mainly in the kidneys and released into the bloodstream in response to anoxia for the stimulation, regulation, and production of erythrocytes.
Urgency	Feeling of a need to void urine immediately.

CONTENT REVIEW

I. Renal system overview
A. Renal structure and function
1. Kidneys are the major organs of the renal system
   a. Cortex—outermost section; contains 85% of nephrons and their surrounding blood supply
   b. Medulla—innermost section; contains portions of the collecting system and renal pyramids
   c. Pelvis—collects and transports urine from kidney to ureter
2. Nephrons are the functional units of the kidney; responsible for urine production; they consist of
   a. Glomeruli—clusters of capillaries surrounded by Bowman's capsule
   b. Tubules—proximal, loop of Henle, distal, and collecting
3. Newborn renal functioning is immature; the system continues to mature during childhood
4. Functions of the renal system
   a. Fluid regulation
   b. Electrolyte balance
   c. Excretion of metabolic wastes
   d. Acid-base balance
   e. Production and control of vitamin D, renin, erythropoietin, and prostaglandins

B. **Renal development**
1. Kidney development begins within the first weeks of embryonic life
2. Kidneys develop from the mesoderm, primary germ layer of the embryo
3. Embryonic development of the kidneys occurs in three stages; the kidney is able to form urine at 10 to 12 weeks' gestation
4. Fetal urine provides a major source of amniotic fluid in the third trimester of pregnancy

C. **Assessment of renal system**
1. Health history
   a. General considerations
      (1) Medications: use of antihypertensives, diuretics
      (2) Urinary characteristics: frequency, color, volume consistent with fluid intake, ease of starting and the force of the stream, ability to empty the bladder
   b. Present problem
      (1) Dysuria
      (2) Urinary frequency
         (a) Change in usual pattern
         (b) Change in volume
         (c) Incontinence
         (d) Change in urinary stream
         (e) Nocturnal enuresis
      (3) Hematuria
         (a) Color—bright red, rusty brown, cola or tea color
         (b) Associated symptoms—pain on voiding; costovertebral or flank pain
      (4) Bleeding
         (a) Parental suspicion of insertion of foreign object; sexual abuse
         (b) Associated symptoms—pain, bladder spasms
      (5) Pain
         (a) Character, location, frequency
         (b) Contributory factors: use of bubble bath, irritating soaps or detergents
      (6) Vaginal discharge
         (a) Relationship to diapers, frequency of change
         (b) Use of lotions, powders
         (c) Possible sexual abuse

        (7) Undescended testicles; testicular mass or pain
        (8) Inguinal area enlargement
            (a) Ability to reduce mass
            (b) Pain in groin
    c. Medical history
        (1) Urinary tract: surgery or injury; congenital anomalies
            (a) Undescended testicles
            (b) Hypospadias; epispadias
            (c) Hydrocele; varicocele
            (d) Ambiguous genitalia
        (2) Major illness
            (a) Kidney disease
            (b) Cardiac disease
            (c) Diabetes mellitus
        (3) Vaginal infections
        (4) Sexually transmitted diseases
    d. Family history
        (1) Kidney disease
        (2) Infertility in siblings
        (3) Hernias
        (4) Congenital anomalies
2. Related laboratory and diagnostic studies (Table 7-1, pp. 257-258)
3. Physical examination
    a. General approach
        (1) Examination of genitalia follows assessment of abdomen while the child is still supine
        (2) In adolescents, inspection of genitalia may be done last
        (3) Use a matter-of-fact approach to decrease anxiety
        (4) Inspection of female genitalia is usually limited to the external structures in childhood
    b. Inspection
        (1) Pubic region
            (a) Hair distribution and configuration
            (b) Surface characteristics of region or external genitalia
        (2) Inguinal hernia present
        (3) Location of urinary meatus
        (4) Vaginal or urethral discharge
    c. Palpation: external genitalia
        (1) Presence of testes with each scrotal sac
        (2) Presence of lesions or growths

D. **Common pediatric medications related to renal/genitourinary function (Table 7-2, pp. 259-264)**

II. Genitourinary tract disorders
A. **Urinary tract infection (UTI)**
1. Description: presence of infection of the upper or lower portion of urinary tract
2. Etiology: escherichia coli and other gram-negative organisms are most often implicated
3. Incidence
    a. Peak incidence for nonstructural UTI is between 2 and 6 years of age
    b. In all ages except neonatal, females have much greater risk for UTI because of shorter urethra
4. Pathophysiology
    a. By location the urinary meatus is in close proximity to the rectum; thus, stool easily contaminates meatus and bacteria ascend into the urethra to the bladder; most common organism is E. coli in females
    b. Urinary stasis is the most critical host factor in development of UTI in older children; urine remaining in the bladder is an excellent medium for bacterial growth
    c. Frequent, prolonged bubble baths may contribute to infections in toddlers, preschoolers, and school-age children
5. Assessment
    a. Assessment findings
        (1) Infancy period
            (a) Dehydration, failure to thrive
            (b) Vomiting
            (c) Irritability
            (d) Foul-smelling urine
        (2) Preschool period
            (a) Fever
            (b) Weak urinary stream
            (c) Abdominal pain—usually suprapubic
        (3) School-age period
            (a) Dysuria
            (b) Frequency
            (c) Urgency
            (d) Change in urinary odor

        (4) Adolescent period
           (a) Dysuria
           (b) Frequency
           (c) Hematuria

  b. Diagnostic studies
        (1) Urine culture to identify bacterial infection
        (2) Intravenous pyelogram to visualize abnormalities in renal structures
        (3) Voiding cystourethrogram reveals anatomic abnormalities that predispose child to UTI

6. Therapeutic management
  a. Medications: antibiotics—penicillins and sulfonamides
  b. Surgical correction of anatomical defect, if present

7. Nursing management
  a. Acute care
        (1) Nursing diagnosis: hyperthermia
        (2) Expected outcome: child's body temperature returns to baseline parameters
        (3) Interventions
           (a) Assess temperature using age-appropriate route q 1 to 2 hours for sudden elevations
           (b) Administer antipyretic, as ordered, for temperatures >102° F
           (c) Provide lightweight clothing and bed linens
           (d) Use tepid sponge bath for 30 minutes; dry each body part after sponging and cover to prevent chilling
           (e) Encourage oral fluid intake
           (f) Use cooling blanket, if appropriate

  b. Home care
        (1) Nursing diagnosis: knowledge deficit
        (2) Expected outcomes
           (a) The parents verbalize knowledge of medication administration, preventive measures for recurrence, and the need for follow-up care
           (b) Child's urine cultures are negative for infectious agent following course of treatment
        (3) Interventions
           (a) Inform parents of the cause of the infection and any contributing factors

        (b) Instruct parents to collect a urine speciman for a culture before and after antibiotic therapy; then usually at monthly intervals for three months, and then at three-month intervals for next six months

        (c) Teach preventive measures: avoid use of frequent, prolonged bubble and tub baths and tight-fitting nonabsorbable clothing; proper feminine hygiene—wiping perineal area from front to back; encourage fluid intake, especially acidic fluids (citrus and cranberry juices); encourage child to void every 2 to 3 hours and to completely empty the bladder with each urination; suggest the use of cotten underwear, especially under pantyhose for teens

        (d) Explain care involved for pre and postdiagnostic procedures that are ordered

  c. Additional nursing diagnoses

    (1) Pain

    (2) Altered urinary elimination

8. Evaluation

  a. Urinary tract infection is eliminated

  b. Child exhibits absence of temperature elevation

  c. Child resumes usual pattern of urinary elimination

B. Vesicoureteral reflux (VUR)

1. Description: condition caused by the back flow of urine from the bladder into the ureters and sometimes into the kidneys (Figure 7-1)

2. Etiology: factors causing

  a. Infection

  b. Congenital malformation

  c. Obstruction

  d. Neurologic dysfunction

3. Incidence: occurs most often in children <5 years of age, before growth alters the renal structures

4. Pathophysiology

  a. Two processes are responsible for increased risk of VUR

    (1) Ureterovesical junction dysfunction

    (2) Voiding dysfunction

  b. Defect graded according to the degree of the upper urinary tract and the effect on lower ureter

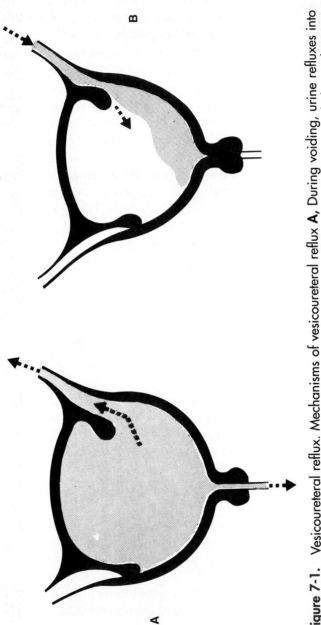
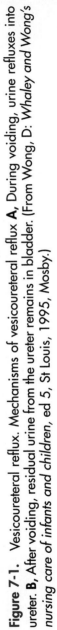

Figure 7-1. Vesicoureteral reflux. Mechanisms of vesicoureteral reflux **A,** During voiding, urine refluxes into ureter. **B,** After voiding, residual urine from the ureter remains in bladder. (From Wong, D: *Whaley and Wong's nursing care of infants and children,* ed 5, St Louis, 1995, Mosby.)

5. Assessment
   a. Assessment findings
      (1) Frequency, urgency, and dysuria
      (2) Nocturia, nocturnal enuresis
      (3) Flank pain, unilateral or bilateral; pain found on side of involvement
      (4) Colic
   b. Diagnostic studies
      (1) Intravenous pyelogram to determine presence of defect
      (2) Voiding cystourethrogram reveals anatomical location of abnormality
      (3) Urine culture and sensitivity indicates presence of infectious agent and specific type of antibiotic therapy
6. Therapeutic intervention
   a. Medications
      (1) Antibiotics to treat organism identified in culture. Example: Ampicillin, sulfisoxazole (Gastrisin).
      (2) Analgesics to control postoperative pain
      (3) Antispasmodics to relax smooth muscle of the bladder and decrease discomfort associated with bladder spasm. Example: oxybutynin chloride (Ditropan).
   b. Surgery—ureteral reimplanation
7. Nursing management
   a. Acute care
      (1) Nursing diagnoses
         (a) Altered urinary elimination
         (b) Risk for injury and infection
      (2) Expected outcome. child establishes normal pattern of elimination
      (3) Interventions
         (a) Assess urine output from indwelling urinary catheter: amount, presence of blood, clots, odor
         (b) Assess indwelling catheter site for presence of redness, swelling, drainage
         (c) Use sterile technique when performing dressing changes, catheter care
         (d) Maintain urinary collection bag below level of bladder; assess tubing often to prevent kinking and obstruction
         (e) Secure catheter to groin or upper thigh to avoid placing tension on catheter

(f) Note the time and amount of the first voiding after indwelling catheter is removed; maximum time to allow is 12 hours
b. Home care
(1) Nursing diagnosis: knowledge deficit
(2) Expected outcomes
(a) Child's urinary elimination pattern will return to within normal limits for the child
(b) Family complies with medication administration regimen and follow-up care
(3) Interventions
(a) Instruct parents to administer antibiotics and the side effects to report, including diarrhea, superinfections, skin rash
(b) Instruct parents on proper technique for obtaining urine specimen for a culture by midstream technique
(c) Inform parents to notify physician if there is a change in the pattern of urinary elimination until a voiding cystourethrogram reveals absence of VUR
(d) Instruct parents on the care of an indwelling urinary catheter, if child is discharged with one in place
(e) Instruct parents to notify physician if the child has signs of infection—cloudy urine, spike in temperature, increased bladder spasms
c. Additional nursing diagnoses
(1) Pain
(2) Hyperthermia
(3) Altered renal tissue perfusion
8. Evaluation
a. Family complies with the administration of the antibiotic regimen
b. Child remains free from further urinary tract infections
c. Normal urinary pattern is reestablished for the child

III. Glomerular disease
A. Acute glomerulonephritis (AGN)
1. Description: an acute autoimmune disorder characterized by an inflammation of the glomeruli that follows an antecedent group-A beta hemolytic streptococcal infection

2. Etiology: occurs 10 to 14 days following upper respiratory infection or otitis media
3. Incidence: peak incidence is between 4 and 7 years of age
4. Pathophysiology
   a. Antigen-antibody complexes damage glomeruli in the basement membrane
   b. Inflammation of the glomeruli occurs and glomeruli become infiltrated with polymorphonuclear leukocytes
   c. Plasma filtration decreases; excess water accumulates and sodium is retained
5. Assessment
   a. Assessment findings
      (1) Puffiness of face—especially periorbital: around the eyes
      (2) Anorexia
      (3) Urine output decreased; urine is cloudy and described as the color of tea or cola
      (4) Irritability, lethargy, headaches
      (5) Abdominal discomfort, vomiting
   b. Laboratory studies
      (1) Urinalysis reveals the presence of protein, hematuria, casts, red and white blood cells; increased specific gravity
      (2) Serum creatinine is increased with impaired renal function; creatinine clearance—most specific test of glomerular dysfunction
      (3) Serum electrolytes monitor for elevations of potassium and phosphate if renal failure occurs
      (4) BUN is increased with impaired renal function
      (5) Antistreptolysin O titer—reveals past streptococcal infection
      (6) Erythrocyte sedimentation rate is increased in presence of any acute inflammatory process
      (7) Throat culture is positive for streptococcal infection at time of inflammation
   c. Complications
      (1) Acute renal failure
      (2) Hypertension
      (3) Hematuria, proteinuria
      (4) Hypertensive encephalopathy
      (5) Nephrotic syndrome

6. Therapeutic management
   a. Medications
      (1) Antibiotics—specific to identified microorganism
      (2) Antihypertensives—with diuretics to treat mild hypertension
   b. Treatments
      (1) Low-sodium diet for children with edema or hypertension
      (2) Restricted potassium and phosphate in diet if renal failure
7. Nursing management (Table 7-3, p. 265): acute/home care
   a. Nursing diagnoses
      (1) Fluid volume excess
      (2) Altered nutrition: less than body requirements
      (3) Activity intolerance
      (4) Risk for infection
      (5) Knowledge deficit
   b. Expected outcomes
      (1) Child's dietary requirements are maintained with adequate fluid balance
      (2) Family verbalizes an understanding of the disease process and follow-up care
8. Evaluation
   a. Child demonstrates stable weight and improved urine output
   b. Family complies with treatment plan, including medication and diet regimine and follow-up care

B. Nephrotic syndrome
   1. Description: clinical condition caused by damage to the glomerular structure of the kidneys with the result of proteinuria and hypoalbuminemia
   2. Etiology: classified according to duration and kidney damage
      a. Minimal change nephrotic syndrome (MCNS)—cause unknown
      b. Secondary nephrotic syndrome—occurs in conjunction with or follows glomerular damage caused by acute glomerulonephritis, collagen diseases, or a drug toxicity
      c. Congenital nephrotic syndrome—caused by a recessive gene
   3. Incidence

   a. MCNS accounts for 80% of diagnosed cases; this is the predominant type of nephrotic syndrome in the preschool child

   b. In the congenital type, death occurs within the first 2 years of life if a kidney transplant is not performed

4. Pathophysiology

   a. In MCNS, a nonspecific illness such as a viral upper respiratory disorder precedes the symptoms by 4 to 8 days

   b. Membrane of glomeruli, usually impermeable to albumin and large proteins, now becomes permeable especially to albumin

   c. The decreased serum albumin causes fluid to accumulate in the interstitial spaces and the body cavities

   d. The resulting hypovolemia stimulates the renin-angiotensin mechanism and the secretion of antidiuretic hormone and aldosterone

   e. Serum cholesterol, phospholipids, and triglycerides are all elevated

5. Assessment

   a. Assessment findings

      (1) Generalized edema: periorbital edema present in morning; abdominal swelling or dependent edema evident in afternoon

      (2) Proteinuria

      (3) Lethargy and irritability

      (4) Abdominal ascites

      (5) Pallor color to skin

      (6) Decreased urine volume; urine opalescent and frothy

   b. Diagnostic procedures

      (1) Laboratory studies

         (a) Urinalysis—reveals massive proteinuria, presence of hyaline casts, RBCs; increased specific gravity

         (b) Serum albumin: decreased

         (c) Serum cholesterol: increased to 450-1500 mg/dl

         (d) Serum phospholipids and triglycerides—elevated

         (e) CBC—reveals increased platelet count as result of hemoconcentration

      (2) Diagnostic studies: renal biopsy—reveals type of nephrotic syndrome and presence of edema from the renal abnormality

6. Therapeutic management

   a. Medications

             (1) Antiinflammatories: prednisone—suppresses clinical manifestations of inflammation; induces remission

             (2) Immunosuppressants: cyclophosphamide (Cytoxan)—for use with children who do not respond to steroid therapy or have frequent relapses

             (3) Diuretics: furosemide (Lasix) in combination with metalozone—used in children with edema that interferes with respiration or causes hypertension

             (4) Antibiotics: penicillin—administered prophylactically or to treat an infection

        b. Treatments—diet: no added salt during periods of severe edema; high-protein, high-calorie diet

      7. Nursing management (see Table 7-3, p. 265): acute/home care

        a. Nursing diagnoses

             (1) Fluid volume excess

             (2) Risk for injury—tissue injury of the skin

             (3) Altered nutrition: less than body requirements

             (4) Activity intolerance

             (5) Knowledge deficit

             (6) Body image disturbance

        b. Expected outcomes

             (1) Child demonstrates no evidence of skin breakdown

             (2) Child gradually resumes normal activities for age as edema subsides

             (3) Parents exhibit knowledge regarding the disease, actions for follow-up procedures, and proper technique of medication administration

      8. Evaluation

        a. Parents implement therapies and follow-up care

        b. Child exhibits decreased edema and resumes age-appropriate activities; no evidence of skin breakdown

IV. Miscellaneous genitourinary disorders

  A. Hypospadias/epispadias

    1. Description: congenital defects involving abnormal placement of the urethral orifice of the penis

    2. Etiology: cause theorized to be multifactorial genetic defect; occurs in intrauterine development with failure of fusion that involves the folds that close the urethra in the penis

    3. Incidence

      a. Epispadias is far less common and occurs in varying degrees of severity

     b. Hypospadias occurs in 1 out of 300 male children; incidence greatest in families with a history of the defect

4. Pathophysiology
     a. Hypospadias—in mild cases the meatus is just below tip of penis; severe cases involve placement on perineal surface between the halves of the scrotum
     b. Severe cases of hypospadias also involve ventral curvature caused by replacement of normal skin with a fibrous band of tissue
     c. Epispadias is often associated with exstrophy of the bladder

5. Assessment
     a. Hypospadias—orifice located below glans penis along ventral surface; may be associated with chordee
     b. Epispadias—urethral orifice located on dorsal surface of penis

6. Therapeutic management: surgical correction for both defects
     a. Hypospadias: urethral lengthening; construction of meatal orifice; chordee release
     b. Epispadias: penile and urethral lengthening; bladder neck reconstruction to establish urinary continence

7. Nursing management
     a. Acute care: preoperative
        (1) Nursing diagnoses
           (a) Anxiety
           (b) Body image disturbance
        (2) Expected outcomes
           (a) Family verbalizes decreased anxiety about defect and surgery
           (b) Child exhibits age-appropriate coping with body image change
        (3) Interventions
           (a) Assess anxiety level of parents and child
           (b) Provide opportunities for parents to discuss the cause of the defect, the possibility of surgical correction, and placement of a urinary indwelling catheter
           (c) Allow parents to verbalize fears and concerns related to procedures and surgery
           (d) Provide opportunities for parents to participate in child's care
           (e) Facilitate the child's expression of feelings and emotions

b. Home care: postoperative
  (1) Nursing diagnosis: altered pattern of urinary elimination
  (2) Expected outcome: child remains free from postoperative complications such as urinary retention, infection after indwelling catheter is removed
  (3) Interventions
    (a) Assess intake and output, urine characteristics
    (b) Provide support and privacy for child during catheter removal and afterwards during attempts to void
    (c) Assess for pain, inability to void, and abdominal distention after catheter removal
    (d) Encourage increased fluid intake
    (e) Teach parents to notify physician of any changes in pattern of urinary elimination once the child is home
c. Additional nursing diagnoses
  (1) Pain
  (2) Risk for infection
8. Evaluation
  a. Child exhibits return of normal urinary elimination pattern after catheter removal
  b. Parents verbalize positive effect of surgical correction with minimal anxiety
  c. Child expresses positive behaviors to cope with effect of surgery

B. **Cryptorchidism**
  1. Description: failure of one or both testes to descend through the inguinal canal into the scrotal sac
  2. Etiology: possible causes of failure to descend
    a. Anatomic obstruction
    b. Testicular dysgenesis
    c. Gonadal hormone deficiency
    d. Genetics
  3. Incidence
    a. Males born before the seventh month of gestation have 100% chance of undescended testes; full-term infants have a 3% occurrence rate
    b. After 1 year of age, the testes do not drop spontaneously

4. Pathophysiology
   a. Testes usually descend down inguinal canal into scrotum during the seventh month of gestation
   b. Possible complications of undescended testes
      (1) Infertility
      (2) Malignant tumors
      (3) Hernias
      (4) Testicular torsion
5. Assessment: examiner does not palpate a small nodular area in each of the testes
6. Therapeutic management
   a. Medications
      (1) Analgesics to control postoperative pain
      (2) Hormones to enhance descent of testes into scrotum
   b. Surgery: orchiopexy performed before 3 years of age
7. Nursing management
   a. Acute/home care
      (1) Nursing diagnoses
         (a) Body image disturbance
         (b) Anxiety
      (2) Expected outcomes
         (a) Family discusses the needed care before and after the correction of the defect including image concerns
         (b) The parents and child exhibit a lowered anxiety level related to surgery and the change of physical attributes
      (3) Interventions
         (a) Assess the parents' and child's level of anxiety
         (b) Provide opportunity for parents to discuss the defect, surgical correction, and possible complications of infertility and testicular cancer
         (c) Provide opportunities for parents to be involved in child's care
         (d) Use age-appropriate activities to teach child about preoperative and postoperative care
         (e) Following surgery, assist parents with a schedule to resume child's activities
         (f) Teach steps of testicular self-examination at postsurgery follow-up visit to parents and child if appropriate

   b. Additional nursing diagnoses
      (1) Pain
      (2) Risk for infection
8. Evaluation
   a. Parents and child exhibit positive comments regarding changes from surgery
   b. Testes are successfully brought down into the scrotum without postoperative complications
   c. The older child and adolescent client demonstrate proper method of testicular self-examination

C. **Wilm's tumor**
1. Description: encapsulated tumor of the kidney
2. Etiology and incidence
   a. Peak incidence is 3 to 4 years of age
   b. Prognosis depends on the stage of the disease at the time of the diagnosis
   c. Often associated with other congenital anomalies
3. Pathophysiology
   a. The tumor originates from the renoblast cells that originate in the renal parenchyma and extend into the surrounding tissues
   b. Metastasis occurs through the blood stream to the lungs, liver, and bone; or by way of the lymphatic system to the lymph nodes
   c. A rapidly growing tumor may cause obstruction to the inferior vena cava or to the intestine
   d. Staging of Wilm's tumor
      (1) Stage 1: tumor limited to one kidney and is surgically excised
      (2) Stage 2: tumor extends beyond the kidney, but is completely excised
      (3) Stage 3: tumors have residual nonhematogenous tumor cells confined to the abdomen
      (4) Stage 4: tumor metastasis to a distant site: the liver, lung, bone, or brain
      (5) Stage 5: involvement occurs in both kidneys
4. Assessment
   a. Assessment findings
      (1) Mass located in the abdomen, deep within the flank
      (2) Pain
      (3) Hematuria

(4) Hypertension

(5) Fever

b. Diagnostic procedures

(1) Laboratory studies

(a) Liver enzymes—elevated ALT, AST, and LDH

(b) Urinalysis determines the presence of hematuria

(c) CBC reveals increased RBC, polycythemia, as tumor secretes more erythropoietin

(2) Diagnostic studies

(a) IVP and abdominal scan detects mass

(b) Renal angiogram reveals extent of renal involvement

(c) Bone marrow aspiration reveals whether involvement extends to the bone marrow

5. Therapeutic management

a. Medications: chemotherapeutic agents—dactinomycin (Actinomycin-D and vincristine for Stage 1 tumors; vincristine and doxorubicin (Adriamycin MDV) combination for other Wilm's tumors

b. Treatments: radiation therapy—may be preoperative or postoperative; for all stages except Stage 1

c. Surgery: tumor removal or resection; total or partial nephrectomy depending on clinical situation

6. Nursing management

a. Acute/home care

(1) Nursing diagnosis: risk for injury

(2) Expected outcome: child remains free of injury related to surgical procedures and treatments

(3) Interventions

(a) Assess vital signs preoperatively and postoperatively

(b) Preoperative: avoid unnecessary palpation of abdominal mass (post a sign at the bedside): palpation tends to spread tumor cells; diapers to be fastened loosely

(c) Monitor bowel sounds postoperatively, usually return in 48 to 72 hours

(d) Assess incision for signs of infection

(e) Assess mucous membranes for signs of breakdown and dehydration

(f) Provide meticulous oral and anal care

           (g) Maintain reverse isolation if leukopenia is present; limit visitors

           (h) Monitor for signs of altered renal function: irritability, elevated BP, headache, weight gain; first sign of renal failure—a decrease in the amount and frequency of voiding

      (4) Nursing diagnosis: anxiety

      (5) Expected outcomes

           (a) Parents express decreased anxiety as they become aware of disease, treatment, and prognosis

           (b) Child exhibits minimal anxious behaviors

      (6) Interventions

           (a) Assess psychological impact on parents following physician discussion of diagnosis

           (b) Provide parents with opportunities to express feelings related to diagnosis

           (c) Provide age-appropriate activities for child to decrease anxiety

           (d) Explore effective coping mechanisms with parents

           (e) Assign consistent caregiver; provide opportunities for parents to participate in child's care

           (f) Provide parents with information regarding community agencies and support groups

  b. Additional nursing diagnoses

      (1) Altered tissue perfusion

      (2) Ineffective family coping

      (3) During chemotherapy and radiation

           (a) Altered bowel elimination

           (b) Altered nutrition: less than body requirements

           (c) Body image disturbance

7. Evaluation

  a. Parents express reduction in anxiety and a positive attitude regarding effects of therapy

  b. Child remains free of complications related to surgery, radiation, and chemotherapy

  c. Child uses opportunities to express anxiety and feelings

Table 7-1. Summary of Major Diagnostic Genitourinary/Renal Tests for Children

Procedure	Purpose	Indications	Developmental Considerations
Intravenous pyelogram (IVP)	Outlines complete renal anatomy Identifies masses Provides information regarding renal integrity	Renal cysts, calculi Kidney stones Difficulty voiding Possible tumors	*Preparation for procedure:* <2 years: NPO after midnight, 8 oz fluid before test >2 years: give cathartic evening before procedure, NPO after midnight
Renal ultrasound	Determines kidney size and shape	Hydronephrosis Cystic kidney disease Neurogenic bladder	*Preparation:* NPO 6 to 12 hr before Sedation for agitated child—chloral hydrate
Scout film (KUB)—kidney, ureters, bladder	Evaluates kidney size Identifies presence of foreign bodies Provides one-dimensional view of renal system	Difficulty voiding Increased BUN, creatinine	*Preparation:* Explanation as for a routine x-ray
Voiding cysto-urethrography	Visualization of bladder, urethra Reveals reflux of urine or bladder emptying problems	Voiding problems Urinary tract infections	*Preparation:* Prepare child for urethral catheterization

Continued.

Table 7-1. Summary of Major Diagnostic Genitourinary/Renal Tests for Children—cont'd

Procedure	Purpose	Indications	Developmental Considerations
Cystoscopy	Provides direct visualization of bladder and lower urinary tract by means of scope inserted via urethra	Bladder and lower-tract lesions	*Preparation:* Child must remain NPO after midnight Children <10 years of age are usually biopsied under general anesthesia
Renal scan	Reveals vascularization and function of kidneys by injection of radio-active isotope	Glomerulonephritis Transplantation rejection Intrarenal masses	*Preparation:* Explanation of procedure and use of low dose of radiation Insertion of IV line Sedation—age appropriate
Renal biopsy	Identifies renal histology by removal of kidney tissue	Distinguishes between types of nephrotic syndromes Hematuris Nephritis	*Preparation:* NPO 4 to 6 hr with test Sedation—age appropriate Children <10 years of age are usually biopsied under general anesthesia

(Modified from Wong, D: *Whaley and Wong's nursing care of infants and children,* ed 5, St Louis, 1995, Mosby.)

Table 7-2. Commonly Used GU/Renal Medications for Children

Classification	Medication	Indications	Route and Dosage	Side Effects	Nursing Implications
Diuretics, loop	Generic: furosemide Trade: Lasix	Edema in renal failure, Nephrotic syndrome, CHF	PO 2 mg/kg q day or BID; Child: may increase by 1 mg/kg day IV 1 mg/kg q day or BID; may increase by 1 mg/kg q 2 hr, not to exceed 6 mg/kg/day	*CNS:* Vertigo, tinnitus, headache, confusion *CV:* Orthostatic hypotension *GI:* Nausea, vomiting, diarrhea *Hepatic:* jaundice, increased liver enzymes *GU:* Profound diuresis, fluid and electrolyte imbalances *Hematology:* Agranulocytosis *Integumentary:* Rash, urticaria	Assess baseline versus vital signs Monitor I&O q 1 hr as necessary Weigh daily Monitor serum electrolytes: Na, K, Cl Monitor blood glucose creatinine, creatinine clearance Assess for hearing loss Monitor BP standing and lying *Parent education:* Administer same time daily with food–don't administer after 3 P.M., to prevent bed wetting Caution child to rise slowly to avoid fainting, dizziness Eat potassium-rich foods

Continued.

259

Table 7-2. Commonly Used GU/Renal Medications for Children—cont'd

Classification	Medication	Indications	Route and Dosage	Side Effects	Nursing Implications
Diuretics, thiazide	Generic: chloroth-iozide Trade: Diuril				Refer to Table 9-1 for information, pp. 252-257
Anticholinergic	Generic: propran-theline Trade: Pro-Banthine	Bladder control Vesicoureteral reflux	PO Child: 1.5 mg/kg/ day in 4 divided doses	*CNS:* Dizziness, headache, insomnia *CV:* Palpitations, tachycardia *GI:* Dry mouth, paralytic ileus *GU:* Urinary retention *Integumentary:* Urticaria, pruritis *Sensory:* Blurred vision, increased 10 p *Other:* Anaphylaxis	Obtain baseline vital signs *Parent education:* Monitor CNS symptoms for indication of overdosage Crush tablet and mix with small amount of food or fluid Sugerless gum or candy will relieve dry mouth Drug may cause blurred vision

Classification	Name	Uses	Dosage	Side Effects	Nursing Considerations
Antihyper-tensive	Generic: hydralazine Trade: Apresoline	Glomerulo-nephritis Chronic renal failure	PO Child: 0.75-1 mg/kg/day in 2-4 doses (initial dose not to exceed 20 mg) IV 1.7-3.5 mg/kg/day in 4-6 divided doses (initial dose not to exceed 20 mg)	*CNS:* Headache, dizziness *CV:* Palpitations, tachycardia *GI:* Nausea, vomiting *GU:* Dysuria *Hematology:* Agranulocytosis *Integumentary:* Rash, flushing	Monitor BP closely (q15 min during IV administration) Assess daily weight, I&O Monitor CBC, electrolytes *Parent education:* Administer same time daily *Have child:* Avoid quick position change Avoid high-sodium foods Avoid OTC products such as cold and allergy medications
Antihyper-tensive	Generic: propranolol Trade: Inderal	Glomerulo-nephritis	Refer to Table 9-1 for information, pp. 252–257		

Continued.

261

Table 7-2. Commonly Used GU/Renal Medications for Children—cont'd

Classification	Medication	Indications	Route and Dosage	Side Effects	Nursing Implications
Antibiotic sulfonamide	Generic: sulfisoxazole Trade: Gantrisin	Urinary tract infections	PO >2 months *Loading* 75 mg/kg or 2 g/m^2 × 1 dose *Maintenance:* 150 mg/kg/ day in equally divided doses q 4-6 hr (maximum dose 6 g/day) IV *Loading:* 50 mg/kg × 1 dose *Maintenance:* 100 mg/kg/ day q 6 hr	*CNS:* Headache, nervousness, seizures *GI:* Nausea, vomiting, diarrhea *GU:* Crystalluria, hematuria *Hematology:* Agranulocytosis, leukopenia *Integumentary:* Rash, urticaria photosensitivity	Assess for previous allergy to sulfonamide Monitor I&O, encourage PO fluids *Parent education:* Shake PO suspension well; may crush tablet Give on empty stomach 1 hr before meals Completion of full course of medication Child to avoid sunlight or use sunscreen if outside

| Antibiotic penicillin | Generic: ampicillin Trade: Omnipen, Amcill | UTI | PO Child >1 month 50-100 mg/kg/day in divided doses q 6–8 hr IV 50-100 mg/kg/day in divided doses q 6-12 hr | *CNS:* Lethargy, convulsions *GI:* Nausea, vomiting, diarrhea *GU:* Vaginitis, monilissis *Integumentary:* Pruritic rash *Hematology:* Anemia, thrombocytopenia *Other:* Anaphylaxis | Assess for previous allergy to penicillin and cephalosporins Assess for symptoms of yeast infections Administer oral ampicillin on empty stomach to facilitate absorption Monitor liver studies Observe for allergic reaction by taking vital signs and checking skin for rash—abdomen usually Administer IV or IM solution within 1 hr of preparation Refrigerate oral suspension and use within 2 weeks *Parent education:* Child should complete entire course of treatment Report diarrhea or rash to physician |

Continued.

Table 7-2. Commonly Used GU/Renal Medications for Children—cont'd

Classification	Medication	Indications	Route and Dosage	Side Effects	Nursing Implications
Antibiotic, sulfonamide	Generic: co-trimoxazole Trade: Bactrim	UTI	PO 40 mg; 8-10 mg/kg/day in divided doses q 12 hr	*CNS:* Lethargy, nervousness *GI:* Nausea, vomiting *GU:* Increased BUN *Integumentary:* Rash, urticaria *Hematology:* Leukopenia, neutropenia *Other:* Stevens-Johnson syndrome —a serious, sometimes fatal, inflammatory disease; characterized by acute onset of fever, bullae on skin, and ulcers on mucous membranes; pneumonia, pain in joints, and prostration are common; may be in response to an allergic reaction to a drug; treatment—bed rest, antibiotics for pneumonia, steroids, analgesics, mouthwashes, sedatives	*Parent education:* Shake suspension well before administration Tablet may be mixed with small amount of food Give on an empty stomach Administer full course of therapy Maintain hydration Protect child from the sun

Table 7-3. Comparison of Acute Glomerulonephritis and Nephrotic Syndrome (Minimal Change)

Renal Disorder	Causative Factor	Assessment Findings	Treatment	Priority Nursing Interventions	Age of Onset
Minimal change nephrotic syndrome (primary)	Infections	Generalized severe edema (anasarca) Massive proteinuria Microscopic or no hematuria Serum protein: decreased Serum lipid: elevated Fatigue Normal or low BP	Prednisone Lasix Salt-poor albumin	*For edema:* Skin care Bed rest *For infection:* Antibiotics *For diet:* Low sodium High protein High potassium	2 to 3 years
Acute post-streptococcal glomerulo-nephritis (AGN)	Immune complex formation	Primary periorbital and peripheral edema Moderate proteinuria Gross or microscopic hematuria Serum potassium: elevated Fatigue Elevated BP	Antibiotics Antihypertensives Transfusions Iron	*For hypertension:* Bed rest Fluid restriction Monitor BP, neurologic status *For diet:* Low-potassium diet	5 to 7 years

REVIEW QUESTIONS

1. A child has been diagnosed with a urinary tract infection. Which statement about appropriate dietary choices should be given to the parents?
   a. The child should drink adequate amounts of water and juices
   b. Carbonated and caffeinated beverages are recommended
   c. Citrus juices are highly effective in eliminating urinary tract infections
   d. No special recommendations should be made

2. A 6-year-old has been diagnosed with acute glomerulonephritis. Considering the diagnosis, the child is most likely to have which of the following symptoms?
   a. Normal blood pressure and diarrhea
   b. Periorbital edema and grossly bloody urine
   c. Severe, generalized edema and ascites
   d. Severe flank pain and vomiting

3. A parent of a 2-month-old infant who was born 8 weeks prematurely is seen at a local clinic. The parent is concerned that the child's testicle is missing. Which of the following information should the nurse provide?
   a. Explain that testes do not descend until 8 months of age
   b. Infants born before the seventh month of gestation have 100% incidence of undescended testes
   c. The testes should have been present in the scrotal sac at birth
   d. Surgical correction will be necessary

4. When performing a physical assessment on an infant with hypospadias with chordee, the nurse should expect which of the following findings?
   a. Bladder exposed with visible urethral openings
   b. Bulge in the scrotal sac
   c. Urethra opens on the dorsal aspect of the penis
   d. Urethra opens on the ventral side of the penis

5. Following surgical correction of hypospadias, the postoperative care plan for a 1-year-old should include which of these measures?
   a. Collection of frequent urine samples
   b. Frequent warm baths
   c. Transillumination of the scrotal sac
   d. Use of restraints to prevent catheter disruption

6. With a medical diagnosis of acute glomerulonephritis, which of these nursing diagnoses should receive priority?
   a. Fluid volume excess
   b. Risk for impaired skin integrity
   c. Risk for injury
   d. Activity intolerance

7. A preschooler is brought to the pediatrician's office because of a fever and very irritable behavior. The child is diagnosed as having a urinary tract infection. A teaching plan should contain which information related to Bactrim administration?
   a. Avoid exposure to the sun when the child is taking Bactrim
   b. Discontinue the medications when the symptoms disappear
   c. Mix the medication with food
   d. The medication will turn the urine orange

8. Before assessing an infant for undescended testes, the nurse should plan to
   a. Allow the child to defecate
   b. Assess vital signs
   c. Palpate the inguinal canals
   d. Warm her hands and the room

9. A child diagnosed with acute glomerulonephritis should be observed for the side effects of hydralazine (Apresoline), which include
   a. Dry mouth, urinary frequency, headaches
   b. Headaches, palpitations, orthostatic hypotension
   c. Hemorrhage, alopecia, seizures
   d. Photosensitivity, palpitations, jaundice

10. The parents of a child with hypospadias are informed that the infant will have a surgical correction when the child reaches the age of 1½ years. The reason for surgery at this age is because
    a. Children will experience less pain
    b. Chordee may be reabsorbed
    c. The child has not developed body image and castration anxiety
    d. The repair is easier before toilet training

ANSWERS, RATIONALES, AND TEST-TAKING TIPS

Rationales	Test-Taking Tips

1. Correct answer: a

Increased fluid intake will dilute concentrated urine. Juices such as apple acidify the urine; bacterial growth is minimized in acidic urine. Caffeinated beverages act as a diuretic and are not a recommended dietary choice. Option *c* is a false statement; juices acidify the urine but are not "highly" effective in eliminating urinary tract infections. Option *d* is a false statement.

Of the given responses, a is the best selection even though the word "adequate" may have distracted you. Adequate in this case may be defined as forcing fluids.

2. Correct answer: b

In acute glomerulonephritis (AGN), decreased plasma filtration results in an excessive accumulation of water and sodium retention within the vascular space. Initial signs unique to children are puffiness of the face, especially around the eyes, and passage of dark-colored urine, which typically indicates blood is present. The blood pressure would be elevated. In AGN, BP is mildly to moderately increased and anorexia is the major GI finding. The findings in option *c* are consistent with nephrotic syndrome. The findings in option *d* are associated with acute urinary tract infections.

In a disease ending in *-itis,* the thought is that the kidney is inflamed and therefore not filtering appropriately. Thus, blood in the urine, and fluid retention are expected. Select response *b*.

3. **Correct answer: b**

Normally the testes develop in the abdomen, from which they descend into the scrotum during the seventh to ninth month of gestation. Therefore, infants born prematurely usually demonstrate undescended testes. Testes may descend as early as 7 months of age. Option *c* is only a true statement for most term infants. The majority of cryptorchid testes will descend spontaneously without a need for surgery. If undescended by age of 1 year, hormonal injections may be given. If unsuccessful, surgery, called orchioplexy, is done. Cryptorchid is a developmental defect characterized by undescended testes in the scrotum.

If you have no idea of the correct response, match the situation in the stem, "premature birth," with the similar idea in one of the responses: response *b*, "infants born before the seventh month of gestation are premature."

4. **Correct answer: d**

Hypospadias is a condition in which the urethral opening is located on the underside of the glans penis or anywhere along the ventral surface of the penile shaft. The sphincters are not defective; thus, incontinence does not occur. Option *a* is a description of exstrophy of the bladder. Hypospadias is a urethral anomaly, and does not describe problems.

Key words to selection of the correct answer are hypospadias and ventral, which indicate the underside of a structure.

located within the scrotal sac. Option *c* is a description of epispadias, in which the sphincters are defective and the child may experience incontinence.

5. Correct answer: d

Hypospadias repair may require urinary diversion to promote optimal healing and maintain patency of the newly formed urethra. In options *a* and *b* the actions are not associated with hypospadias correction. Option *c* is an assessment technique to identify scrotal anomalies; it has no purpose in this client.

Use a general knowledge approach for the care of a postoperative client to select response *d*. Prevention for accidental removal of tubes and lines is important.

6. Correct answer: a

Regular assessment of intake and output and body weight is essential to monitor the overall fluid balance and the progression of the disease process. Edema associated with AGN is primarily periorbital and peripheral in the hands and feet. Skin care is a major consideration of nephrotic syndrome in which edema is severe and generalized (called anasarca). Fatigue is associated with nephrotic syndrome.

Since the kidney is responsible for fluid and electrolyte balance, a priority nursing diagnosis would be addressing fluid abnormalities.

7. Correct answer: a

Sulfonamides produce photosensitivity, the development of a rash, and

If you have no idea of the correct response, match the medication, Bactrim, in the stem with the

urticaria with exposure to
the sun. The child should
avoid exposure to ultraviolet
light and sunlight. As with
other antibiotics, this
medication should be
administered for the entire
course of therapy, not only
until symptoms disappear.
The sulfonamides should be
administered with adequate
fluids (at least 8 ounces
with each medication
administration). Option *d* is
a side effect of Pyridium
(phenazopyridine
hydrochloride), a urinary
"analgesic" that soothes
the mucosa of the urethra
so burning on urination
is eliminated.

same in the response; choose
response *a*.

8. Correct answer: d

This action decreases the
possibility of cremasteric
reflex, which causes testes to
be pulled back into the
inguinal canal. The actions in
options *a* and *b* are not
relevant to undescended
testes assessment. The action
in option *c* is part of the
assessment activity during
the examination for
undescended testes.

Use common sense to select the
correct response. Assessment of
the testicles requires a palpation
technique in which the client's skin
is exposed to room air and the
temperature of the nurse's hands.

9. Correct answer: b

Apresoline is a direct
vasodilator that acts to relax
peripheral vascular smooth
muscles, resulting in
vasodilation, decreased BP,

Identify that apresoline is an
antihypertensive; a side effect
would be hypotension. Select
response *b* based on this
knowledge. In fact, any

and headache. Direct vasodilation produces side effects related to reflex activity of the sympathetic nervous system: palpitations from the decreased preload. The side effects in the other options are not consistent with apresoline administration.

antihypertensive medication has the potential side effect of orthostatic hypotension. Clients are educated to rise slowly from a lying to a standing position by sitting for 3 to 5 minutes before standing.

10. **Correct answer: c**

At this young age there is a decreased risk of psychological trauma associated with genital surgery. Option *a* is a false statement: chordee, a fibrous band of tissue, is released as part of surgical repair. Toilet training does not influence the ease of surgical repair.

Common sense will guide you to eliminate option *a*; pain does not vary by age. Also eliminate option *d,* since toilet training begins around 18 to 24 months with bowel first then bladder training. Of the two remaining options, *b* and *c*, "go with what you know" and select *c*. Avoid selecting option *b* if you don't know to what it pertains.

Nursing Care of Children with Musculoskeletal Disorders

STUDY OUTCOMES

After completing this chapter, the reader will be able to do the following:

▼ Differentiate between various congenital skeletal defects.

▼ Describe the therapeutic management and the nursing care of a child with scoliosis.

▼ Outline the plan of care for a child with juvenile rheumatoid arthritis.

▼ Describe the nursing care of a child with osteomyelitis.

▼ Differentiate between the manifestations of cerebral palsy and muscular dystrophy.

▼ Describe the etiological factors that contribute to fractures in childhood.

KEY TERMS

Denis-Browne splint	Splint used for the correction of talipes equinovarus (clubfoot) composed of a curved bar attached to the soles of high-topped shoes; it is equipped with wing nuts allowing abduction of each foot to be individualized; it is commonly applied nightly in late infancy after casting and manipulation have effectively reduced the deformity.
Diaphysis	Shaft of a long bone; consists of a tube of compact bone enclosing the medullary cavity.
Epiphyseal plate	Thin layer of cartilage between the epiphysis (the head of the long bone), which is a secondary bone-forming center, and the shaft of the bone; the new bone forms along the plate.
Frejka splint	Corrective device consisting of a pillow that is belted between the legs of a baby born with dislocated hips to maintain abduction and articulation of the head of the femur with the acetabulum.
Pavlik harness	Device used for congenital dislocated hip for infants less than 6 months of age.
Talipes	Refers to deformities that involve the foot and ankle; usually congenital.

CONTENT REVIEW

I. Musculoskeletal system overview

    A. Review of structure and function

        1. Skeletal system

           a. Skeleton is composed of 206 bones, which determine the framework and the body size

               (1) Bones are classified according to shape: long, short, flat, irregular

               (2) Bones have proximal and distal diaphyses that provide sites for muscle and ligament attachment and lend support to the bone

               (3) The site where bones are attached is called a joint, which provides mobility and stability to the skeleton

               (4) Ligaments are fibrous connective tissue that connect bones to each other and provide support to joints between the bones

      b.   The skeleton lies within the muscles and the soft tissues; it has two divisions
          (1)   Axial skeleton—composed of bones that make up longitudinal axis of body
          (2)   Appendicular—includes bones of upper and lower extremities
      c.   Functions of skeletal system
          (1)   Support for body
          (2)   Protection of vital organs and spinal cord
          (3)   Movement: locomotion
          (4)   Storage for minerals
          (5)   Hematopoiesis in red bone marrow mainly in the long bones
  2. Muscular system
      a.   Makes up 25% of infant's body weight
      b.   Muscles classified as voluntary or involuntary
          (1)   Skeletal muscles are voluntary and controlled by conscious effort
          (2)   Cardiac and smooth muscle are involuntary and contract independently of conscious effort
      c.   Tendons are connective tissue between a muscle and the bone to which it is attached
      d.   Function of muscular system
          (1)   Movement
          (2)   Posture
          (3)   Heat production during contraction

B. Development of musculoskeletal system
  1. The musculoskeletal system is derived from the mesoderm germ layer, it is developed after the third week of conception
  2. Through infancy and childhood, the long bones increase in length as a result of proliferation of cartilage at the epiphyses
  3. The timing of bone growth and ossification adheres to a specific sequence in childhood
  4. Bone growth is completed at about 20 years of age when the last epiphysis closes

C. Assessment of musculoskeletal system
  1. Related laboratory and diagnostic studies (Table 8-1, p. 295)
  2. Health history
      a.   General considerations
          (1)   Exercise: extent, type, frequency, stress on specific joints, participation in organized sports

   (2) Nutrition: amount of calcium, vitamin D, and protein

   (3) Medications: muscle relaxants, antiinflammatory agents

  b. Present problem

   (1) Joint, muscular, or skeletal complaints: character, precipitating factor, efforts to treat, presence of growth spurt

   (2) Injury: mechanism of injury, pain, and swelling

   (3) Developmental milestones: fine and gross motor skills appropriate for age

  c. Medical history

   (1) Trauma to the nerves, soft tissue, bones, joints

   (2) Surgery—skeletal or muscular

   (3) Skeletal deformities or congenital anomalies

  d. Family history: congenital anomalies, scoliosis, rheumatoid arthritis or osteoarthritis

 3. Physical examination

  a. Inspection

   (1) Skeleton and extremities

    (a) Alignment

    (b) Symmetry of body parts

    (c) Size

   (2) Skin and subcutaneous tissues over muscles and joints

    (a) Color, ecchymosis

    (b) Swelling, masses

   (3) Contralateral muscles

    (a) Size

    (b) Symmetry

    (c) Spasms

  b. Palpation of bones, joints, and muscles for

   (1) Muscle tone

   (2) Heat

   (3) Tenderness, swelling, pain

   (4) Crepitus

  c. Test joint range of motion

  d. Test strength of muscles

 D. **Musculoskeletal medications (Table 8-2, pp. 296-299)**

II. Musculoskeletal disorders

 A. **Congenital defects**

  1. Congenital dislocated hip

   a. Description: orthopedic congenital disorder involving femoral head, acetabulum, or both

b. Etiology and incidence
   (1) Increased incidence with breech delivery
   (2) Causes
      (a) Fetal positioning
      (b) Cerebral palsy
      (c) Meningocele
      (d) Arthritis
   (3) Left hip is more commonly involved
c. Pathophysiology
   (1) Condition ranges from a mild lateral displacement of the hip to a complete dislocation of the femoral head from the acetabulum
   (2) Subluxation, or incomplete dislocation of the hip, is the most common type
d. Assessment
   (1) Assessment findings
      (a) Asymmetry of the skin folds on the inner side of thigh with child in prone position
      (b) Shortening of the affected leg
      (c) Positive Ortolani's sign—a click or popping sensation felt by examiner when a selected technique is used to evaluate range of motion of hips
      (d) Waddling gait in older child
   (2) Diagnostic studies
      (a) Pelvic x-ray—difficult to interpret in newborns, since ossification of femoral head does not occur until 3 to 6 months of age
      (b) Pelvic ultrasound
e. Therapeutic management
   (1) If diagnosed early, the hip joint may be maintained with a Frejka pillow sprint, or a Pavlik harness for infants up to 6 months of age
   (2) Traction and/or casting is used with older children
f. Nursing management: acute/home care
   (1) Nursing diagnoses
      (a) Risk for injury
      (b) Alteration in skin integrity
   (2) Expected outcome: correct position for femur and acetabulum is maintained without skin breakdown

        (3) Interventions

           (a) Assess infant for signs of hip dysplasia

           (b) Assess neurovascular status of lower extremities

           (c) Apply Pavlik harness to maintain abduction; apply Frejka pillow splint as ordered

           (d) Demonstrate for parents correct application and removal of harness or other treatment devices along with skin inspection

        (4) Additional nursing diagnoses

           (a) Impaired physical mobility

           (b) Altered growth and development

           (c) Anxiety

           (d) Knowledge deficit

    g. Evaluation

        (1) Child regains appropriate hip position without injury or skin breakdown

        (2) Parents return demonstrate correct technique for application of Pavlik harness or other treatment devices

2. Congenital clubfoot (talipes equinovarus)

    a. Description: orthopedic condition involving adducted forefoot, inwardly tilted heel, and plantar flexion of the ankle

    b. Etiology and incidence

        (1) Unilateral clubfoot is more common than bilateral clubfoot

        (2) Occurs as single defect or in association with other disorders or chromosomal anomalies

        (3) Cause unknown; boys more commonly affected

    c. Pathophysiology

        (1) Foot usually assumes a normal position in utero in the seventh month; arrested development has tendency to result in rigid deformity

        (2) Abnormal intrauterine positioning is more likely to result in a more flexible deformity

    d. Assessment

        (1) Assessment findings

           (a) Foot pointed inward and downward

           (b) Fixed positioning of foot or ankle

           (c) Inability to return foot and ankle into alignment

        (2) Diagnostic study: radiographic examination of the foot

   e. Therapeutic management

        (1) Serial casting to gradually manipulate the foot into a normal position; the cast is changed weekly after manual manipulation

        (2) Denis-Browne splint employed to maintain alignment following serial casting

        (3) Surgery—tendonotomy for the more severe forms

   f. Nursing management: acute/home care

        (1) Nursing diagnoses

           (a) Risk for injury

           (b) Knowledge deficit

        (2) Expected outcomes

           (a) Parents demonstrate the correct techniques for use of corrective devices

           (b) Child maintains the correct positioning of the feet without circulatory complications

        (3) Interventions

           (a) Assess the type of deformity and related treatment

           (b) Assess neurovascular status of the lower extremities

           (c) Inform parents of the stages of corrective treatment, as indicated by physician

           (d) Instruct parents in the manipulation procedure, the application of Denis-Browne splint as directed by physician

           (e) Teach parents the care of the infant in a cast

        (4) Additional nursing diagnoses

           (a) Impaired physical mobility

           (b) Pain

           (c) Impaired skin integrity

           (d) Altered growth and development

3. Evaluation

        (1) Child attains maximum use of affected foot and ankle without circulatory complications

        (2) Parents readily participate in long-term medical regimen

B. Disorders related to musculoskeletal growth
1. Legg-Calvé-Perthes disease
   a. Description: disorder characterized by interruption of vascular supply to proximal femoral epiphysis
   b. Etiology and incidence
      (1) Exact causes unknown; the following factors have been thought to be involved: hormones, trauma, infection, and genetics
      (2) Occurs most often in boys between the ages of 3 and 10, with a peak age of 6 years
      (3) Occurs with equal frequency in the right and left hips; bilateral occurrence is rare
   c. Pathophysiology
      (1) Cycle of pathology includes avascular necrosis, revascularization, necrotic bone resorption, and then living bone replacement
      (2) Process occurs over period of 3 to 4 years
   d. Assessment
      (1) Assessment findings
         (a) Pain, often radiating to the groin, thigh, or knee
         (b) A limp observed during ambulation
         (c) Decreased weight bearing on the affected side
      (2) Diagnostic studies
         (a) CT scan and MRI to evaluate femoral head involvement for pathology identification
         (b) Arthrography to determine shape of the femoral head
         (c) Bone scan to determine degree of epiphyseal involvement
   e. Therapeutic management
      (1) Medications: nonsteroidal antiinflammatories
      (2) Medical: non–weight-bearing bracing with abduction orthosis, serial casting
      (3) Surgery—osteotomy of the pelvis or proximal femur
   f. Nursing management: acute/home care
      (1) Nursing diagnoses
         (a) Risk for injury
         (b) Risk for impaired skin integrity
      (2) Expected outcomes
         (a) Head of acetabulum is maintained within acetabulum on affected side

        (b) Parents demonstrate proper application of orthopedic devices and techniques of neurovascular assessment

     (3) Interventions

        (a) Assess symptoms of disease process: limp, frequent need for rest periods

        (b) Assess pain: location, severity, duration

        (c) Assess range of motion noting any limitations with abduction and external rotation

        (d) Demonstrate for parents the care of the prescribed orthopedic device

        (e) If child is casted, apply principles of cast care (refer to nursing management: fractures, p.293)

        (f) Teach parents the use of devices, pertinent neurovascular assessment, pain management, and skin care

     (4) Additional nursing diagnoses

        (a) Impaired physical mobility

        (b) Anxiety

        (c) Altered growth and development

  g. Evaluation: child attains full range of motion of hip with a minimized deformity of femoral head and acetabulum with no skin breakdown

2. Scoliosis

  a. Description: lateral curvature of the spine, most commonly affecting the thoracic area

  b. Etiology and incidence

     (1) Classified as two basic types

        (a) Structural—results from congenital deformity of the spinal column

        (b) Functional—usually occurs secondarily to another preexisting problem such as unequal leg length or poor posture

     (2) Majority of structural scoliosis cases are idiopathic, unknown cause

     (3) Other causes that may contribute

        (a) Trauma

        (b) Neuromuscular disorders: muscular dystrophy; cerebral palsy

     (4) Most often occurs in adolescent girls during their growth spurts

   c. Pathophysiology
- (1) A rotary deformity caused by rotation of the vertebrae that results in physiological changes in the spine, chest, and pelvis
- (2) Curves rapidly progress during periods of rapid growth; they continue until skeletal maturity is achieved

   d. Assessment
- (1) Assessment findings
  - (a) Asymmetrical scapulae
  - (b) Asymmetrical shoulders, hips, and breasts
  - (c) Lateral S-shaped curvature of spine; localized lordosis
- (2) Diagnostic studies
  - (a) Anteroposterior/lateral x-ray of spine reveals curvature of spine and the degree of curvature
  - (b) Scoliometer reveals deformity while child is in a forward-bending position with arms held above the head

   e. Therapeutic management
- (1) Nonsurgical
  - (a) Milwaukee Brace—for curvatures of 20 to 40 degrees; must be worn 23 hours per day; can be removed one hour for bathing
  - (b) Exercises—to prevent atrophy of spinal and abdominal muscles
  - (c) Electrical stimulation—causes the muscles to contract at regular intervals, which causes the spine to straighten; used with mild to moderate curvatures
- (2) Surgical: performed when the nonsurgical methods are unsuccessful in halting progression of the curvature
  - (a) Traction is used before surgery in severe curvatures
  - (b) Spinal fusion is performed to halt progressive worsening of curvature; various instrumentations are used to internally stabilize the spine
    - (i) Harrington rod
    - (ii) Lugue segmental
    - (iii) Dwyer
    - (iv) Cotrel-Dubousset

   f. Nursing management: acute/home care
- (1) Nursing diagnosis: impaired physical mobility

      (2) Expected outcomes

         (a) Child demonstrates correct posture

         (b) Child remains free of complications of immobility

      (3) Interventions

         (a) Nonsurgical management

            (i) Assess for degree of impaired mobility

            (ii) Assess posture with encouragement for correct posture

            (iii) Teach child and parents exercises to decrease spinal curvature or refer to physical therapy

            (iv) Instruct family in correct use and care of a Milwaukee brace including: the brace must be worn 23 hours per day; removal of the brace is allowed for 1 hour to allow for hygiene and skin care; massage the bony prominences and monitor for areas of skin breakdown; eventually the brace will be worn only at night

         (b) Postsurgical management

            (i) Promote adequate pulmonary functioning: encourage periodic deep breathing and keep child well hydrated

            (ii) Maintain child's body in alignment

            (iii) Log roll from side to side every 2 hours with two pillows between legs and one pillow under the head

            (iv) Perform passive range of motion exercises as directed by physician

            (v) Encourage participation in ADLs when possible

      (4) Nursing diagnosis: body image disturbance

      (5) Expected outcome: child adapts to limitations imposed by corrective appliance or other devices

      (6) Interventions

         (a) Assess child for concerns regarding the wearing of orthopedic devices, any lifestyle limitations, and social interaction difficulties with peer group

         (b) Provide opportunities for participation in activities allowed

         (c) Provide opportunities for participation in ADLs, application and removal of brace, care of skin

        (7) Other nursing diagnoses
           (a) Altered growth and development
           (b) Risk for impaired skin integrity
           (c) Impaired breathing pattern

    g. Evaluation
        (1) The child actively participates in the orthopedic regimen
        (2) The child participates in appropriate family and social activities within the given restrictions of the condition

C. Inflammatory and infectious disorders

  1. Juvenile rheumatoid arthritis (JRA)

    a. Description: chronic inflammatory disease affecting the joints; juvenile onset is diagnosed before 16 years of age

    b. Etiology and incidence
        (1) Cause unknown; familial tendency
        (2) Two peak ages of onset: between 2 and 5 years and between 9 and 12 years
        (3) Types of JRA (Table 8-3, p. 300)
           (a) Pauciarticular—involving less than five joints
           (b) Polyarticular—involving five or more joints
           (c) Systemic onset—involves arthritic symptoms, elevated temperature, rash, and dysfunction of other organs such as the heart, lungs, eyes, and organs located within abdominal cavity

    c. Pathophysiology
        (1) Synovial inflammation results in joint effusion and erosion and then gradual destruction of the joint cartilage
        (2) Muscle spasm initially causes limited movement; later ankylosis or contracture is the cause of limited movements
        (3) Exacerbation of symptoms of JRA can be caused by surgery, infection, and injury

    d. Assessment
        (1) Assessment findings (see Table 8-3, p. 300)
           (a) Temperature elevations to 102° F orally; primarily in late afternoon or evening
           (b) Stiffness, swelling, loss of motion in the affected joints

    (2) Diagnostic procedures
       (a) Laboratory studies
           (i) Erythrocyte sedimentation rate (ESR)— may or may not be elevated depending on degree of inflammation
          (ii) Rheumatoid factor—positive in pauciarticular
         (iii) Antinuclear antibodies—positive in 40% of cases
         (iv) CBC—reveals leukocytosis in acute systemic JRA
       (b) Diagnostic studies: joint x-ray—reveals widened joint spaces; inflammation and osteoporosis at the affected joint sites

e. Therapeutic management: medications
    (1) Nonsteroidal antiinflammatory drugs—aspirin, ibuprofen to relieve fever, inflammation, and pain
    (2) Slower acting antirheumatic drugs—gold, penicillamine inhibit formation of collagen, inhibit prostaglandin synthesis
    (3) Corticosteroids—prednisone to suppress inflammation; used sparingly for short periods of time because of undesirable side effects
    (4) Cytotoxic drugs—cyclophosphamide (Cytoxan), methotrexate—used when other antiinflammatory agents have not been effective

f. Nursing management: acute/home care
    (1) Nursing diagnosis: chronic pain
    (2) Expected outcome: child verbalizes relief of pain with a reduction in the inflammation
    (3) Interventions
       (a) Assess severity of joint pain, as well as quality, location, onset, duration
       (b) Assess limitations of mobility imposed by the pain and degree of deformity
       (c) Administer antiinflammatories as ordered; evaluate their effectiveness
       (d) Assist to a position of comfort: support the painful joints when moving
       (e) Provide opportunities for use of nonpharmacologic pain relief methods: imagery, diversional activities, relaxation techniques

              (f)   Apply splints as ordered

              (g) Apply warm compresses to affected areas; whirlpool and paraffin dips as ordered

      (4) Nursing diagnosis: self-care deficit

      (5) Expected outcome: child demonstrates ability to independently carry out ADLs

      (6) Interventions

              (a) Assess current level of functioning with ADLs

              (b) Provide opportunities for independent behavior; assist as necessary

              (c) Provide necessary equipment and assistive devices to perform ADLs

              (d) Consult occupational therapy for adaptive equipment; reinforce self-care techniques

              (e) Inform parents of child's need for independence and progression in ADLs

      (7) Additional nursing diagnoses

              (a) Altered growth and development

              (b) Fatigue

              (c) Ineffective family coping

  g. Evaluation: child exhibits positive actions to maintain ADLs with minimal help from parents

2. Osteomyelitis

  a. Description: infection of the bone tissue; usually involves the long bones and is preceded by infection or trauma in another part of the body

  b. Etiology and incidence

      (1) Occurs more commonly in males; age affected is between 5 to 14 years

      (2) Although any organism may cause this infection, staphylococci is the major cause in older children; hemophilus influenza is the major causative agent in younger children

      (3) Sources of infection

              (a) Exogenous—from an outside source, as a result of a wound, fracture, surgical contamination

              (b) Hematogenous—preexisting focus of infection is a skin abrasion, impetigo, tooth abscess, infected burn, or otitis media

      (4) Predisposing factors: poor nutrition, hygiene, and physical condition

c. Pathophysiology
    (1) Organisms invade the bone metaphysis; the infectious process leads to bone destruction and an abscess formation
    (2) Pressure from the abscess causes lifting of the periosteum
    (3) Infection spreads under the periosteum, and additional bony necrosis and granulation occur; sinus cavities form between the dead bone and the skin surface

d. Assessment
    (1) Assessment findings
        (a) Pain in affected area
        (b) Fever
        (c) Warmth over area
        (d) Irritability
        (e) Guarding or unwillingness to move affected limb
    (2) Diagnostic procedures
        (a) Laboratory studies
            (i) Positive blood culture
            (ii) CBC—indicates leukocytosis
            (iii) Erythrocyte sedimentation rate—elevated
        (b) Diagnostic study: x-ray—reveals soft tissue swelling

e. Therapeutic management
    (1) Medications: long-term IV antibiotics
    (2) Treatments
        (a) Splint affected area; bed rest
        (b) Surgical incision and drainage of area; drainage tube insertion such as penrose
        (c) Closed-tube antibiotic irrigation of bone

f. Nursing management: acute/home care
    (1) Nursing diagnosis: pain
    (2) Expected outcome: child verbalizes relief of pain and associated symptoms
    (3) Interventions
        (a) Assess site for pain with movement, guarding
        (b) Use age-appropriate pain-rating scale
        (c) Monitor vital signs
        (d) Administer analgesic as ordered
        (e) Immobilize limb; support affected extremities with pillows at 30 degrees elevation
        (f) Apply warm compresses to affected area

         (g) Provide age-appropriate diversional activities as tolerated

      (4) Additional nursing diagnoses

         (a) Risk for injury

         (b) Hyperthermia

         (c) Impaired physical mobility

         (d) Anxiety

         (e) Diversional activity deficit

  g. Evaluation: child exhibits behaviors that control pain

D. Neuromuscular dysfunction: cerebral palsy (CP)

  1. Description: nonprogressive motor function disorder characterized by impaired movement and posture; usually is associated with abnormal or premature birth and intrapartal asphyxia

  2. Etiology and incidence

    a. Most common permanent physical disability of childhood

    b. Other factors associated with CP

      (1) Congenital and perinatal infections

      (2) Congenital brain anomalies

      (3) Intrauterine ischemia

    c. Classification of CP is based on the nature and distribution of the neuromuscular dysfunction

      (1) Spastic CP—characterized by upper motor neuron type of muscular weakness

      (2) Dyskinetic CP—characterized by abnormal involuntary movements

      (3) Ataxic CP—caused by cerebellar defect; characterized by nonprogressive failure of muscle coordination and irregular muscle action

      (4) Mixed-type cerebral palsy—characterized by combination of spasticity and athetosis: slow, writhing involuntary movements of the extremities

      (5) Rigid, tremor, and atonic types—uncommon types of CP

  3. Pathophysiology

    a. Caused by permanent neurologic lesions ranging from gross brain malformations to vascular occlusion, neuron loss, and laminar degeneration

    b. Cerebral anoxia is the most significant factor in brain damage

    c. In the dyskinetic type, basal ganglia damage results in uncontrollable involuntary movement; it is aggravated by stress

4. Assessment
   a. Assessment findings: general
      (1) Delayed gross motor development
      (2) Abnormal motor performance—unilateral hand use at 6 months of age
      (3) Abnormal posturing—evident with spastic CP
      (4) Persistence of primitive infantile reflexes and reflex hyperactivity
   b. Associated disabilities
      (1) Mental retardation
      (2) Seizures
      (3) Attention deficit–hyperactivity disorder
      (4) Sensory impairment: strabismus, hearing loss
5. Therapeutic management
   a. Medications: diazepam and other medications for spasticity
   b. Assistive devices for mobility and communication
   c. Physical and occupational therapy
   d. Surgery—tenotomy of the adductors with lengthening of the tendons and hamstring release
   e. Dorsal rhizotomies or ventral thalamotomies—to improve the ability to walk
6. Nursing management: acute/home care
   a. Nursing diagnosis: self-care deficit—feeding, hygiene, toileting
   b. Expected outcome: child performs ADLs, as tolerated
   c. Interventions
      (1) Encourage child to participate in ADLs according to condition with referral to occupational therapy
      (2) Adapt clothing and grooming aids to enable child to dress and groom independently
      (3) Adapt feeding utensils (wide-bowled spoon) to allow self-feeding; provide finger foods
      (4) Assist parents to toilet train child
   d. Nursing diagnosis: risk for injury
   e. Expected outcome: child remains free of injury
   f. Interventions
      (1) Assess child's environment for potential risks
      (2) Provide safety measures: side rails up when in bed, provide safety helmet, padded furniture, restraints when in chair or moving vehicles
      (3) Adhere to seizure precautions if history of seizures
      (4) Provide adequate rest periods between activities

      b.   Additional nursing diagnoses
         (1)   Impaired physical mobility
         (2)   Impaired skin integrity
         (3)   Impaired verbal communication
  7. Evaluation
      a.   Child engages in self-care activities to maximum ability
      b.   Child remains safe within the environment

E. Muscular dysfunction: pseudohypertrophic (Duchenne) muscular dystrophy (MD)

  1. Description: most severe and common form of MD, resulting in muscle wasting and weakness
  2. Etiology and incidence
      a.   Transmitted as sex-linked recessive gene
      b.   Affects males, most commonly between the ages of 3 and 5
      c.   Death occurs 10 to 15 years after the diagnosis, usually from respiratory complications
  3. Pathophysiology
      a.   Bilateral wasting of the voluntary muscles
      b.   Hypertrophy of the muscles; replacement of muscle tissue with fatty deposits and connective tissue
  4. Assessment
      a.   Assessment findings
         (1)   Progressive muscle weakness, wasting, and contractures
         (2)   Calf muscle hypertrophy
         (3)   Waddling gait and lordosis
         (4)   Difficulty in rising from a sitting or supine position
         (5)   Frequent falls, clumsiness
         (6)   Developmental delays
      b.   Complications
         (1)   Contractures
         (2)   Disuse atrophy
         (3)   Infection
         (4)   Obesity
         (5)   Cardiac failure
      c.   Diagnostic procedures
         (1)   Laboratory study: serum enzyme studies reveal increased CPK with muscle deterioration
         (2)   Diagnostic studies
            (a)   Electromyogram reveals decreased electrical activity in affected muscles

        (b)   Muscle biopsy reveals muscle degeneration and replacement with fatty tissue

5. Therapeutic management
   a. Medications: antibiotics for respiratory infection
   b. Treatments: physical therapy—range of motion, casting, bracing; occupational therapy for ADLs
   c. Surgery: release of contractures
6. Nursing management: acute/home care
   a. Nursing diagnoses
      (1) Impaired gas exchange
      (2) Ineffective airway clearance
   b. Expected outcome: child maintains optimal gas exchange with absence of infections
   c. Interventions
      (1) Assess respiratory function, breathing pattern
      (2) Evaluate strength of respiratory muscles
      (3) Reinforce diaphragmatic breathing techniques taught by respiratory therapist
      (4) Position to ease respiratory effort; suction as needed
   d. Nursing diagnosis: impaired physical mobility
   e. Expected outcome: child maintains optimal physical mobility
   f. Interventions
      (1) Assess strength of muscles; mobility
      (2) Assess body alignment
      (3) Monitor changes in CPK as indicator of muscle deterioration
      (4) Offer physical and occupational therapy to reinforce range of motion and ADL program
   g. Additional nursing diagnoses
      (1) Risk for impaired skin integrity
      (2) Impaired verbal communication
      (3) Body image disturbance
7. Evaluation
   a. Child remains ambulatory as long as possible without skin breakdown
   b. Child remains free of respiratory infection

F. **Fractures**
1. Description: break in bone associated with a fall or other trauma; classified according to the tissue injury
   a. Simple or closed: fracture that has no open wound
   b. Compound or open: fracture in which the bone breaks through the skin and results in an open wound

      c. Comminuted fracture in which the bone is splintered or crushed

2. Etiology and incidence

      a. Greenstick fracture is the most common type in children <3 years of age

      b. Other fracture types occurring in childhood

         (1) Open or closed

         (2) Buckle (torus) impact injury that is characterized by a projection near the metaphysis

         (3) Complete fracture that involves the entire cross-section of the bone

      c. Common fracture sites for children

         (1) Forearm

         (2) Clavicle

         (3) Femur

         (4) Tibia

         (5) Fibula

      d. Motor vehicle accidents are a frequent cause of bone injury at all ages, particularly between 4 and 7 years of age

3. Pathophysiology

      a. Growth in length occurs at the epiphyseal plate

      b. Children's bones are more pliable and porous than adults' bones, which allows the bones to bend, buckle, or result in greenstick fracture

      c. Fractures occur as a result of a direct or indirect force on the bone, repeated stress on a bone, or pathologic conditions

      d. Healing of bone is more rapid in children: bone healing takes 1 week for every year of life up to 10 years of age

4. Assessment

      a. Assessment findings

         (1) Pain

         (2) Tenderness

         (3) Swelling

         (4) Limited movement

      b. Diagnostic procedures

         (1) Laboratory studies

            (a) Serum enzymes—creatine phosphokinase, alkaline phosphatase, AST (SGOT), LDH— elevated according to amount of damage

            (b) WBC count—elevated neutrophils

         (2) Diagnostic study: x-ray—to reveal a fracture at an injury site

    c. Complications
- (1) Circulatory impairment
- (2) Nerve damage
- (3) Compartment syndrome
- (4) Volkmann (ischemic) contracture—a serious, persistent flexion contracture of the forearm and hand caused by ischemia
- (5) Damage to epiphyseal plate
- (6) Infection
- (7) Pulmonary emboli
- (8) Kidney stones

5. Therapeutic management
- a. Medications: analgesics, narcotic and nonnarcotic for pain control
- b. Treatments: casting or traction, skin or skeletal, to immobilize and realign affected area
- c. Surgery: open reduction, with or without pinning

6. Nursing management
- a. Nursing diagnosis: pain
- b. Expected outcome: child verbalizes reduced pain
- c. Interventions
    - (1) Assess child for pain and discomfort using age-appropriate pain scale
    - (2) Immobilize and elevate affected extremity; reposition unaffected parts for comfort
    - (3) Administer analgesic or muscle relaxant as ordered
    - (4) Apply ice to site for first 48 hours to decrease swelling if ordered
    - (5) Encourage relaxation techniques
- d. Nursing diagnosis: altered peripheral tissue perfusion
- e. Expected outcome: child exhibits a reduced risk of neurovascular complications
- f. Interventions
    - (1) Assess site distal to the fracture every 1 to 2 hours until stable, noting color (pallor or cyanosis), sensation, capillary refill, movement, pulse equality, temperature
    - (2) Allow cast to dry, turning q 2 hours, using palm of hand to handle cast
    - (3) Elevate casted extremity on a pillow
    - (4) Remove articles with small parts from the area to prevent child from putting them into the cast
    - (5) Petal cast if rough edges exist

          (6) Outline area of drainage on cast with pen; place date and time nearby

          (7) Clean plaster cast with vinegar and water, fiberglass cast with mild soap and water

          (8) Provide quiet age-appropriate activities

          (9) Provide range of motion to unaffected extremities

        (10) Teach parents cast care and assessment of neurovascular status

        (11) Massage skin at cast edges to prevent skin breakdown; do not use lotions or powder, which soften skin

        (12) Reinforce techniques of crutch walking

        (13) Inform parents how to apply a sling

  g. Additional nursing diagnoses

      (1) Risk for injury

      (2) Impaired physical mobility

      (3) Risk for infection

7. Evaluation

  a. Child verbalizes a decrease in pain

  b. Parents and child demonstrate proper techniques of cast care and/or use of assistive devices

Table 8-1. Summary of Major Musculoskeletal Diagnostic Procedures for Children

Procedures	Purpose	Indications	Developmental Considerations
X-ray	Isolate and identify musculoskeletal pathology	Suspected child abuse Bone fractures	Infants and young children may need sedation or restraints to be immobilized during x-ray
Computerized axial tomography (CAT) scan	Diagnose bone pathology Determine size and location of masses, tumors	Soft tissue masses or bone tumors	Sedation may be necessary for infants and young children Age-appropriate explanations should be provided before procedure
Magnetic resource imaging (MRI)	Evaluate pathological changes in musculoskeletal system	Spinal or joint structural defects Bone deformities	Child and family need thorough instructions including the need for immobility and the expected noises during the procedure, loud clicking
Arthroscopy	Provide direct visualization of joints by means of endoscope	Joint damage Ligament damage Synovial disease	Child must be kept NPO after midnight Procedure done under general or spinal anesthesia
Bone scan	Detect pathology of musculoskeletal system	Bone pain Osteomyelitis Metastatic bone disease	Explanation must be provided regarding injection of radioactive isotopes Sedation may be necessary to immobilize child Child must void before procedure

Table 8-2. Commonly Used Musculoskeletal Drugs for Children

Classification	Medication	Indications	Route and Dosage	Side Effects	Nursing Implication
Antibiotic	Generic: clindamycin Trade: Cleocin	Used to treat gram-positive bacterial infections Osteomyelitis	PO >1 month 8-25 mg/kg/day in 3 to 4 divided doses IM, IV <1 month 15-20 mg/kg/day in 3 divided doses >1 month 15-40 mg/kg/day in 3 to 4 divided doses	*GI:* Nausea, vomiting, diarrhea, pseudomembranous colitis *CV:* Hypotension, cardiac arrest *Hematology:* Leukopenia, eosinophilia *Integumentary:* Rash, pruritus, urticaria, anaphylaxis	Assess for previous allergies to this drug Administer PO on empty stomach Assess for signs of superimposed infection, especially yeast Monitor renal studies for protein and blood *Parent education:* Teach parents importance of entire course of medications Teach the need to inform physician of any side effects, especially diarrhea

Classification	Drug	Uses	Dosage	Side Effects/Adverse Reactions	Nursing Considerations
Antibiotic	Generic: nafcillin, oxacillin Trade: Nafcil	Used to treat penicillinase—producing staphylococcus aureus Osteomyelitis	PO 50-100 mg/kg/day q 6 hr in equally divided doses IM, IV 100-200 mg/kg/day q 12 hr (IM), q 4 hr or q 6 hr (IV)	CNS: Lethargy, anxiety, depression GI: Nausea, vomiting, diarrhea GU: Vaginitis, hematuria, proteinuria Integumentary: Rash, pruritus Hematology: Thrombocytopenia, leukopenia	Assess for previous allergies to this drug Administer PO on an empty stomach Dilute IV medication according to label instructions IM injection painful—give Z-track if possible
Antibiotic	Generic: penicillin G potassium Trade: Deltapen	Gram-positive and gram-negative organisms Osteomyelitis	PO Child (<12 years) 25,000-90,000 U/kg/day in 6 divided doses IM, IV 25,000-50,000 U/kg/day in 4 divided doses	CNS: Lethargy, anxiety, depression GI: Nausea, vomiting, diarrhea GU: Vaginitis, moniases Hematology: Anemia, bone marrow depression Integumentary: Rash	Assess for previous allergies Assess liver, blood, and renal studies Administer PO on an empty stomach with full glass of water Stress importance of medication compliance

Continued.

Table 8-2. Commonly Used Musculoskeletal Drugs for Children—cont'd

Classification	Medication	Indications	Route and Dosage	Side Effects	Nursing Implication
Anti-inflammatory (nonsteroidal)	Generic: indomethacin Trade: Indocin	Juvenile rheumatoid arthritis (JRA) Degenerative joint disease	PO 2 to 14 years 1.5-2.5 mg/kg/day in 3 to 4 doses, not to exceed 4 mg/kg/day	*CNS:* Dizziness, headache *CV:* Fluid retention, hypertension, palpitations *GI:* Heartburn, nausea, vomiting *Respiratory:* Dyspnea *Hepatic:* Jaundice *GU:* Polyuria *Sensory:* Blurred vision	Assess prior allergy to this drug, ASA, or other nonsteroidal medications Administer with food *Parent education:* Administer with food, as directed Avoid other OTC medications, unless prescribed Report to physician: rash, flu-like symptoms, visual changes
Anti-inflammatory (steroidal)	Generic: prednisone Trade: Cortalone Deltasone	Suppress inflammatory responses and reactions JRA	PO 0.14 to 2 mg/kg/day q 6 hr in equally divided doses	*Sensory:* Increased intra-ocular pressure *CNS:* Euphoria, psychotic behavior *CV:* Edema, HTN *GI:* Nausea, vomiting *GI:* Irritation	Obtain baseline height and weight Monitor serum electrolytes *Parent education:* Weigh child daily and monitor I&O Administer with food Do not withdraw medication quickly

Anti-inflammatory (steroidal) —cont'd	*Integumentary:* Impaired wound healing, facial redness *Hematology:* Thrombocytopenia *MS:* Suppressed bone growth *Endocrine:* Cushing's states	Child should wear medical alert bracelet Report sudden weight gain to physician Inform any health-care provider that child is on this medication Observe for signs of infection, since child has increased risk

Table 8-3. Clinical Manifestations of Subtypes of Juvenile Rheumatoid Arthritis

Subtype	Age of Onset	Joints Involved	Systemic Symptoms	Laboratory Findings
Systemic onset	1 to 3 years 8 to 10 years	Any	Rheumatoid rash Polyarthritis Fever, malaise	Elevated: Rheumatoid factor (RF) Erythrocyte sedimentation rate (ESR) Antinuclear antibody (ANA) positive
Pauciarticular	Type I: mostly female, <10 years of age	Lower extremities—knee, ankle, sacroiliacs	Iridocyclitis—inflamation of the iris and ciliary body causing redness of sclera adjacent to corner of eye	ANA positive ESR elevated
Polyarticular	Throughout childhood	Any, usually small joints	Minimal systemic signs Low-grade fever Malaise Rheumatoid nodules	Type I: RF positive Type II: RF negative ESR elevated

REVIEW QUESTIONS

1. A parent has been given instructions about a Pavlik harness to be worn by the infant with congenital hip dysplasia. Which of these statements by the parent indicates that there is an understanding of the instructions?
   a. "We plan to remove the harness for 1 hour per day"
   b. "We'll make follow-up appointments for harness readjustment"
   c. "We must maintain the legs in an adducted position"
   d. "We can remove the harness for diaper changes"

2. When performing a physical assessment of a 12-year-old client, the nurse should expect which of these findings related to scoliosis?
   a. Asymmetry of the shoulders, back, and waist
   b. Convex angulation in thoracic area
   c. Concave curvature of lumbar spine
   d. Malformation of vertebrae

3. An 18-month-old boy is scheduled for application of a plaster cast to correct a clubfoot. The postoperative plan should include which of the following measures?
   a. Elevate the cast above the level of the heart
   b. Handle cast with fingertips
   c. Reposition the child every 2 hours
   d. Spray the cast with acrylic

4. A preadolescent boy has juvenile rheumatoid arthritis. He has been ordered to receive sodium salicylate (aspirin), 650 mg, QID. During the course of drug administration, the nurse should assess for which of the following?
   a. Constipation, irritability, and headache
   b. Diarrhea, periorbital edema, and gastric distress
   c. Nausea, vomiting, and tinnitus
   d. Edema, hearing loss, and choking

5. A 9-year-old girl has been brought to the emergency department following an automobile accident and is diagnosed with a femoral fracture. Which of these goals should receive priority in the child's care?
   a. Adequate nutrition will be maintained
   b. Infection will be prevented
   c. Disturbance in body image will be reduced
   d. Pain will be reduced

6. The school nurse would screen a female adolescent for scoliosis by instructing her to
   a. Bend forward at the waist and allow upper extremities to dangle
   b. Lie prone on an examination table
   c. Sit on a chair and raise shoulders
   d. Stand with shoulders placed against the wall

7. Which of these approaches would most likely encourage an overweight adolescent diagnosed with juvenile rheumatoid arthritis to comply with a weight-loss program?
   a. Allow parents to select diet from low-calorie menu
   b. Encourage the client's input with meal planning
   c. Require daily weigh-ins
   d. Require client to eat meals alone

8. Which of these assessments of a child with a cast for correction of a clubfoot needs to be reported?
   a. Cast has not dried in 2 hours
   b. Color change and cool skin proximal to cast
   c. Moves toes and capillary refill is <3 seconds
   d. Rough edges on the cast

9. An adolescent must wear a Milwaukee brace. To promote the teen's optimal functioning, which of these actions should the nurse take?
   a. Discourage participation in ADLs
   b. Inform the teen that the brace may be removed for several hours daily for comfort
   c. Teach appropriate application, removal, and care of brace
   d. Teach non–weight-bearing techniques

10. A parent asks why her infant must wear a Pavlik harness. The nurse responds that the purpose of this device is to
    a. Provide comfort and support
    b. Shorten the limb on the affected side
    c. Maintain the femur within the acetabulum
    d. Provide outward displacement of the femoral head

ANSWERS, RATIONALES, AND TEST-TAKING TIPS

Rationales	Test-Taking Tips

1. Correct answer: b

The infant should be examined by the practitioner before any adjustment is attempted. It is important to ensure that the hips are in correct placement before the harness is resecured. Harnesses may or may not allow for removal for bathing. A Pavlik harness is used to maintain the hip in abducted position. Diapering may be accomplished without harness removal.

Eliminate response *a,* since no reason for removal is given. Eliminate response *c,* to keep legs adducted, recalling that the client has the abductor pillows to keep the hip in the joint after hip joint replacement. The same approach would be used with this condition. Eliminate response *d,* since response *b* is more appropriate; when harnesses are applied removal is typically minimal.

2. Correct answer: a

This is a classic finding in scoliosis, which is identified when the client (facing away from the examiner) is asked to raise both arms and bend forward at the waist, allowing the arms to dangle. Another way to describe the findings is an unequal height of the hips or shoulders. Option *b* is a description of kyphosis, which is a more common finding in older women with osteoporosis. Option *c* is a description of lordosis, which may be found in children and middle-age men who have gained weight in the abdominal area. Scoliosis involves spinal curvature, not malformation of the vertebrae that make up the spinal column.

Remember that *s*coliosis is an *S*-shaped curvature of the spine that results in *a*symmetry of the back structures.

3. Correct answer: c

Turning the child every 2 hours will help to dry the cast evenly. Drying can take up to 72 hours if traditional plaster cast materials are used. Casted extremities should be elevated on a pillow to increase venous return and will not, in all cases, be elevated above the heart especially in an 18-month-old client. Another way to implement appropriate elevation is to raise the distal joint higher than the proximal joint of the extremity. The cast should be handled by the palms of the hands to prevent indenting the cast, which creates pressure areas. Option *d* is not a nursing responsibility.

If you narrowed the responses to *a* and *c*, reread the stem to note that the age of the client is 18 months. Therefore, response *c* is the better selection, since this age of child is more active and would be quite difficult to keep in a position in which the feet are above the heart. Also recall that a cast needs to be repositioned to facilitate drying, especially within the first 24 to 48 hours.

4. Correct answer: c

Characteristic side effects associated with salicylates involve the GI system, resulting from the action of salicylates on the emetic center of the medulla and the local irritation on the gastric mucosa. Hearing problems include hearing loss and tinnitus (ringing in the ears), when high doses are taken. Not all of the findings in the other options are side effects associated with salicylates.

Read the responses vertically to help clarify the correct response. For example: constipation, diarrhea, nausea, and edema. Of these responses, eliminate *a* and *b,* since they relate to lower GI; ASA more likely affects upper GI. Eliminate option *d* since choking is unrelated to ASA administration. So select response *c* as the correct answer.

5. Correct answer: d

Control of pain, hemorrhage, and edema is the priority in caring for the child with a femur fracture. Option *a* is not an immediate priority for a child with a fracture. If a surgical incision is present, the goal in option *b* would likely be included in the child's plan of care. Option *c* is a psychosocial need and part of planning for home care.

As with similar acute injuries, provision for comfort is the priority in any client's care.

6. Correct answer: a

Structural asymmetry, one hip or shoulder higher than the other, is observed posteriorly when the child bends from the waist unsupported with the arms. The positions in the other options do not reveal any asymmetrical skeletal formation.

If you have no idea of the correct response, cluster responses *b, c,* and *d* under the category of static positioning; select response *a,* which is a dynamic positioning.

7. Correct answer: b

Client participation in meal planning to include likes and dislikes will increase the likelihood of compliance. The teen is capable of making appropriate choices, with guidance; this action fosters independence. Weight reduction progress should be measured by weekly or biweekly weigh-ins. The approach in option *d* prevents socialization at mealtimes, which is often important to teens.

The best answer is the one that includes the client's input and actions.

8. Correct answer: b

Any discoloration of a casted extremity or change in the neurovascular status needs to be reported. A cast made of traditional materials may take up to 72 hours to dry. The findings in option *c* indicate a normal neurovascular status. Raw edges of the cast can be protected by a petaled edge applied with tape by the nurse, without physician involvement.

The key words are "color change" and "cool skin proximal." These words indicate abnormalities that must be reported.

9. Correct answer: c

When a brace must be worn, the use and care of the orthopedic appliance is explained to facilitate correction of the defect. Return demonstrations should be done before the parents and adolescent go home. Adolescents should participate maximally in ADLs to meet their physical developmental needs and tasks. The Milwaukee brace may be removed for 1 hour daily for bathing and at no other time. The action in option *d* is not appropriate intervention for an adolescent with a brace.

Eliminate responses *a* and *d* since they are false statements. Reread the question and note the key words "to promote optimal functioning." Select response *c* since it more adequately answers the question. Response *b* presents only one aspect of optimal functioning.

10. Correct answer: c

The Pavlik harness, along with gravity, works the hip into a more abducted position with the proximal femur centered in the acetabulum. It is used

An approach is to remember that a more common finding in infants is hip displacement; make the educated guess to select response *c*.

to correct congenital hip displacement. Positioning of the femoral head is the primary purpose, not comfort or support. Leg shortening on the affected side is a finding consistent with congenitally dislocated hips. The abduction device in option *d* maintains the femur in the acetabulum.

▼ ▼ ▼ ▼ ▼ ▼ ▼ ▼ ▼   ▼ ▼ ▼

Nursing Care of Children with Endocrine Disorders

STUDY OUTCOMES

After completing this chapter, the reader will be able to do the following:

▼ Describe the functions of the endocrine system.
▼ Describe the functions of the major endocrine glands.
▼ Discuss the nursing diagnoses and the interventions commonly needed for children with selected endocrine dysfunction.
▼ Describe the psychosocial implications for the family and the child newly diagnosed with diabetes mellitus.
▼ Distinguish between a hyperglycemic and hypoglycemic reaction.

KEY TERMS

Enuresis	Incontinence of urine, especially while sleeping.
Gland	Any one of many organs in the body, comprised of specialized cells that secrete or excrete materials not related to their ordinary metabolism; some lubricate, others produce hormones, and others such as the spleen and lymph take part in the production of blood components.
Hormone	Complex chemical substance produced in one part or organ of the body that initiates or regulates the activity of an organ or group of cells in another part of the body; secretion of hormones by the endocrine glands is regulated by other hormones, neurotransmitters, and a negative feedback system.
Hyperglycemia	Greater than normal amount of glucose in the blood; in diabetes mellitus it is best diagnosed by the glucose tolerance test; normal test results: (fasting) 70 to 115 mg/dl; (30 min and 1 hour) <200 mg/dl; (2 hour) <140 mg/dl; (3 and 4 hours) 70 to 115 mg/dl.
Hypoglycemia	Less than normal level of glucose in the blood; best tested by a random serum glucose; glucose level <50 mg/dl.
Insulin	Naturally occurring hormone secreted by the beta cells of the islands of Langerhans in the pancreas in response to increased levels of glucose in the blood.
Negative feedback	To decrease the function in response to a stimulus; for example, the follicle-stimulating hormone decreases as the amount of circulating estrogen decreases.

CONTENT REVIEW

I. **Endocrine system overview**
    A. **Review of structure and function**
        1. Glands of the endocrine system are located throughout the body (Table 9-1, pp. 320-322)
            a. Hypothalamus
            b. Pituitary

      c. Thyroid

      d. Parathyroid

      e. Pancreas

      f. Adrenal

      g. Ovary

      h. Testes

2. Endocrine glands produce and secrete hormones directly into the bloodstream in response to specific signals (see Table 9-1, pp. 320-322)

3. Major processes controlled by the endocrine glands include growth, maturation, metabolic function, and reproduction

4. Regulation of hormone levels is controlled by feedback systems

5. Endocrine problems occur from hyperfunction or hypofunction of the glands

B. Development of endocrine system

1. Endocrine glands are well developed at birth; however, their functions are immature

2. Thyroid gland develops during the seventh to fourteenth week of intrauterine development

3. The pituitary gland's gross features are recognizable by the end of the third month of intrauterine life

4. Parathyroid glands are forming during the fifth week of fetal development from the dorsal wings of the third and fourth pharyngeal pouches

5. Ovaries are distinguishable from testes by the sixth week of gestation

6. The pancreas contains the islets of Langerhans, which are endocrine tissues arising from parenchymatous pancreatic tissues during the third month of fetal life

C. Assessment of endocrine function

1. Health history

      a. General

         (1) Past growth measurements, heights and weights of family members

         (2) Endocrine disorders in relatives

      b. Nutrition

         (1) Timing and content of meals

         (2) Recent changes in appetite or weight

         (3) Plotting of growth patterns on growth chart

      c. Elimination

         (1) Change in usual pattern of elimination

         (2) Characteristics of urine and stool

    d. Activity
        (1) Changes in child's endurance and participation in physical activity
        (2) Frequency of physical activity
  2. Related laboratory and diagnostic studies (Table 9-2, p. 322)
  3. Physical examination
    a. Obtain vital signs and compare to norms for age
    b. Obtain accurate physical measurements and plot on growth chart: height, weight, and head circumference
    c. Head and neck
        (1) Inspect for facial anomalies, prominence of the eyes, asymmetry
        (2) Presence of thyroid masses or enlargement
    d. Chest: breast development is noted for males and females and compared to Tanner stage
    e. Pelvic region
        (1) Female genitalia changes: enlarged clitoris, labial fusion
        (2) Male genitalia inspected for penis size, location of urethra, testicular development and size, scrotal development
        (3) Distribution and configuration of pubic hair
    f. Integument
        (1) Hair distribution
        (2) Texture
        (3) Acne
        (4) Hyperpigmentation or depigmentation

D. Commonly used medications for endocrine disorders (Table 9-3, pp. 323-325)

II. Insulin-dependent diabetes mellitus (IDDM): type I diabetes

A. Description: metabolic disorder characterized by inability of pancreas to secrete insulin

B. Etiology and incidence
  1. Cause unknown; however, affected individual is believed to have a genetic predisposition resulting in autoimmune response
  2. A viral infection may act as the precipitating factor
  3. This most common metabolic disorder has a peak incidence between 5 and 7 years of age and during early adolescence

C. **Pathophysiology**
   1. With insulin deficiency, glucose is unable to enter the cell; this results in hyperglycemia
   2. When glucose is unavailable for cellular metabolism, the body uses other sources of energy such as fats and protein; this results in ketoacidosis
   3. Insulin deficiency also increases the effects of counter-regulatory hormones: epinephrine, glucagon, cortisol, and growth hormone

D. **Assessment**
   1. Assessment findings
      a. Three cardinal symptoms: polydipsia, polyphagia, polyuria
      b. Weight loss
      c. Hyperglycemia
      d. Yeast infections
      e. Abdominal discomfort
      f. Dehydration
      g. Fatigue
      h. Enuresis
   2. Complications
      a. Diabetic ketoacidosis
      b. Coma
      c. Microvascular changes: neuropathy, retinopathy, nephropathy
      d. Limited joint mobility in some cases
   3. Laboratory studies
      a. Blood glucose—levels >120 mg/dl in fasting specimen; >200 mg/dl in random sample; >300 mg/dl in ketoacidosis
      b. White blood cell count—increased with predominantly polymorphonuclear lymphocytes
      c. Ketones—increased in blood and urine

E. **Therapeutic management**
   1. Medication
      a. Regular and NPH insulin administered subcutaneously as two or more doses daily; dosage is individualized based on blood glucose monitoring
      b. Portable infusion pump is an alternate method of delivering continuous infusion
      c. Most commonly, 60% to 75% of daily dose is administered before breakfast; remainder is taken before the evening meal

      2. Nutrition—consistent meal plan encouraged

      3. Exercise—part of total diabetic management plan, since blood glucose levels decrease with exercise; therefore, insulin needs decrease

F. Nursing management

    1. Acute care

      a. Nursing diagnosis: altered nutrition: less than body requirements

      b. Expected outcome: child maintains nutritional requirements adequate to support growth and development, while diabetes is controlled

      c. Interventions

        (1) Assess for signs of hyperglycemia or diabetic ketoacidosis

        (2) Assess blood glucose level (normal: 70 to 110 mg/dl)

        (3) Administer insulin as ordered

        (4) Provide appropriate diet with calories that balance with energy expenditure

        (5) Offer meals on time; provide between-meal snacks

        (6) Instruct family in dietary planning while emphasizing adequate caloric intake according to age; discuss importance of proper meal times

        (7) Consult dietician for diet education

        (8) Offer food lists for free foods and exchanges according to four food groups

        (9) Assist in sample meal planning

        (10) Provide opportunities for exercise

    2. Home care

      a. Nursing diagnosis: knowledge deficit

      b. Expected outcomes

        (1) Child and family demonstrate compliance with treatment regimen: insulin therapy, blood testing, exercise, diet planning

        (2) Child and family verbalize knowledge regarding disease pathology, activity/exercise needs, dietary and medication requirements

      c. Interventions

        (1) Assess cognitive abilities and readiness to learn

        (2) Provide quiet environment; limit sessions to 15 to 20 minutes; use a variety of teaching methods: videos, comic books

(3) Explain definition of diabetes, need for diet restrictions, and importance of daily exercise
(4) Instruct the family on proper technique of insulin administration, handling and storage, rotation of injection sites
(5) Instruct family on method of testing blood glucose (Chemstrips or Accu-check system)
(6) Define hypoglycemia and causes; teach symptoms and actions to treat (Table 9-4, p. 326)
(7) Define hyperglycemia and causes; teach symptoms and actions to treat (see Table 9-4, p. 326)
(8) Reinforce the need for routine follow-up for the prevention of complications of diabetes
(9) Discuss importance of record keeping: insulin, test results, responses to diet and exercise; take to follow-up visits
(10) Inform parents that food intake depends on activity level and insulin intake

d. Additional nursing diagnoses
(1) Risk for injury
(2) Risk for impaired skin integrity
(3) Risk for fluid volume deficit
(4) Ineffective family coping

G. **Evaluation**
1. Child maintains a daily blood glucose level of <120 mg/dl and >60 mg/dl
2. Family and child comply with medical regimen for control of diabetes
3. Child and family demonstrate correct technique of insulin administration and blood glucose testing
4. Child has minimal episodes of extreme glucose levels

III. Hypothyroidism

A. **Description: common endocrine disorder resulting from inadequate production of thyroid hormone**
B. **Etiology and incidence**
1. Classification of causes
a. Congenital—examples: autoimmune thyroiditis, hypopituitarism, thyroid dysgenesis
b. Acquired—examples: thyroidectomy, irradiation, dietary deficiency of iodine, thyroiditis

2. Hypofunction of the thyroid gland is far more common in childhood than is hyperfunction
3. Hyperthyroidism, a condition characterized by a high concentration of thyroid hormone that increases metabolic function, is found mainly in adolescents with Graves' disease
4. Congenital hypothyroidism is the most common cause of primary hypothyroidism; occurs in 1 out of 2500 live births
5. Diseases such as tuberculosis and mumps may contribute to the development of thyroiditis

C. **Pathophysiology**
1. Development and prognosis of the disease depends on the type of defect, age of onset, and severity of deficiency
2. Thyroid gland secretions
    a. Thyroxine (T_4): regulates metabolic rate; promotes mobilization of fats and gluconeogenesis; plays important role in bone, teeth, and brain development
    b. Triiodothyronine (T_3): same as T_4
    c. Thyrocalcitonin: regulates calcium and phosphorus metabolism; contributes to ossification and bone development; inhibits bone resorption—loss of calcium from the bone
3. Complications
    a. Retarded skeletal growth
    b. Delayed eruption of teeth
    c. Mental retardation
    d. Ataxia
    e. Strabismus

D. **Assessment**
1. Assessment findings
    a. Infants
        (1) Slow growth
        (2) Facial appearance—small forehead, flattened nasal bridge, large protruding tongue
        (3) Hoarse cry
    b. Children
        (1) Dry skin
        (2) Sparse, brittle hair
        (3) Nonpitting myxedema
2. Diagnostic procedures
    a. Laboratory studies
        (1) Thyroid hormones by radioimmunoassays—decreased T_3, T_4, and TSH, thyroid stimulating hormone from the anterior pituitary

        (2) Protein-bound iodine: increases after age 2
          months
    b. Diagnostic studies: thyroid scan—to determine size,
      location, and shape of gland; radioactive iodine uptake by
      thyroid is scanned

E. Therapeutic management: medications
  1. Hormones—levothroxine sodium as replacement for
    decreased or absent thyroid function
  2. Vitamins—calcitrol to ensure adequate calcium levels during
    periods of growth

F. Nursing management
  1. Acute care
    a. Nursing diagnosis: impaired physical mobility
    b. Expected outcome: child maintains optimal mobility within
      disease and developmental limitations
    c. Interventions
        (1) Assess therapeutic response to the administration of
          thyroid replacement, including linear growth and
          activity level
        (2) Monitor for signs of drug toxicity: irritability,
          nervousness, tachycardia, tremors, diarrhea
        (3) Schedule follow-up for monitoring of serum levels
          of T_3, T_4
  2. Home care
    a. Nursing diagnosis: knowledge deficit
    b. Expected outcome: family exhibits adequate knowledge
      of disease along with compliance of medication
      regimen
    c. Interventions
        (1) Assess family's knowledge of the disorder and
          replacement therapy goals
        (2) Instruct parents about administration of thyroid
          replacement, side effects, necessity of periodic
          monitoring of serum levels
        (3) Inform parents to expect gradual improvement in
          activity levels
  3. Additional nursing diagnoses
    a. Risk for impaired skin integrity
    b. Altered nutrition: less than body requirements
    c. Constipation
    d. Sensory-perceptual alterations
    e. Fatigue

G. Evaluation
   1. Family complies with daily thyroid replacement regimen
   2. Child displays improved function and activity level without signs of hypothyroidism

IV. Hypopituitarism

A. **Description: decreased or inadequate secretion of pituitary hormones**
B. **Etiology and incidence**
   1. Hypopituitarism occurs as a result of the following
      a. Tumors in pituitary or hypothalamic region
      b. Irradiation
      c. Infection
      d. Head trauma
   2. Most commonly affects boys
C. **Assessment**
   1. Assessment findings
      a. Retarded growth pattern
      b. Appears younger than chronologic age
      c. Delayed eruption of permanent teeth
      d. Delayed sexual development
      e. Premature aging later in life
   2. Diagnostic procedures
      a. Laboratory study: serum growth hormone level to reveal absent or decreased growth hormone
      b. Diagnostic studies
         (1) Review of child's growth in height and weight
         (2) Skeletal survey
         (3) X-rays of wrist and skull to determine bone infection and presence of tumor
         (4) CT scan to localize lesion
D. **Therapeutic management**
   1. Medications: growth hormone replacement—biosynthetic form
   2. Surgical: removal of tumor, if present
E. **Nursing management**
   1. Acute care
      a. Nursing diagnosis: knowledge deficit
      b. Expected outcome: parents demonstrate skill in administration of growth hormone
      c. Interventions
         (1) Discuss diagnosis and long-term treatment with family

            (2)   Discuss need for frequent injections of growth hormone

            (3)   Teach parents correct technique of injection of growth hormone

  2. Home care

      a. Nursing diagnosis: self-esteem disturbance

      b. Expected outcome: child verbalizes positive feelings about self

      c. Interventions

            (1)   Discuss with family and child the probability that child will eventually reach adult height and that puberty is delayed by 1 to 2 years

            (2)   Encourage family to treat child at appropriate level for age

            (3)   Provide emotional support for child and family

      d. Additional nursing diagnoses

            (1)   Impaired social interaction

            (2)   Fear

            (3)   Altered parenting

F. **Evaluation**

  1. Family complies with growth hormone replacement regimen

  2. Child achieves adult height

  3. Child participates in group activities with peers

Table 9-1. Summary of Major Endocrine Hormones and their Actions

Gland/Hormone	Actions
Anterior pituitary	
Growth hormone (GH)	Promotes bone and soft tissue growth and protein synthesis Facilitates fat mobilization for energy
Thyroid-stimulating hormone (TSH)	Promotes growth and secretory activity of thyroid Promotes growth and development
Adenocortico-tropic hormone (ACTH)	Stimulates growth and secretory activity of adrenal cortex (cortisol, androgens)
Follicle-stimulating hormone (FSH)	Development of seminiferous tubules and spermatogenesis in males Follicle malleation and estrogen stimulation in females
Leutenizing hormone (LH)	Stimulates secretion of progesterone by corpus luteum in females Causes rupture of follicle and release of mature ova
Prolactin	Stimulates milk secretion Provides maintenance of corpus luteum during pregnancy
Posterior pituitary	
Antidiuretic hormone (ADH)	Regulates osmolarity and water volume Increases permeability of kidneys' collecting ducts
Oxytocin	Stimulates uterine contraction Stimulates letdown reflex—release and flow of breast milk
Thyroid gland	
Thyroxine (T_4) and triodothyro-nine (T_3)	Influences metabolism and bone, teeth, and brain growth Influences lipid and carbohydrate metabolism
Calcitonin	Stimulates bone development and ossification

Table 9-1. Summary of Major Endocrine Hormones and their Actions—cont'd

Gland/Hormone	Actions
Parathyroid gland	
Parathyroid hormone (PTH)	Influences calcium and phosphorous metabolism Regulates phosphorous excretion Regulates calcium reabsorption from bone, blood, and intestines
Pancreas	
Insulin (beta cells)	Promotes glucose, protein, and lipid metabolism Promotes transport of glucose across cell membrane Promotes hepatic storage of glucose
Glucagon (alpha cells)	Counters regulatory hormone to insulin with epinephrine, growth hormone, and glucocorticoid Increases blood glucose from stimulation of breakdown of glycogen stores in liver Decreases protein synthesis and lipolysis
Adrenal cortex	
Mineralcorticoid ▼ Aldosterone	Causes sodium reabsorption by renal tubes and potassium excretion
Sex hormones ▼ Androgens	Influences secondary sex characteristics in boys and girls
Glucocorticoids ▼ Cortisol ▼ Cortisone	Facilitates fat, protein, and carbohydrate metabolism Acts as antagonist to insulin Causes an antiinflammatory action Promotes gluconeogenesis Influences protein and fat catabolism Promotes retention of sodium and water with a loss of potassium
Adrenal medulla	
Calecholamines ▼ Epinephrine ▼ Norepinephrine	Increases contractility and excitability of heart muscle Increases basal metabolic rate Increases blood flow to muscles, brain, and viscera Regulates glycogenolysis, lipolysis Stimulates alpha and beta receptors

Continued.

Table 9-1. Summary of Major Endocrine Hormones and their Actions—cont'd

Gland/Hormone	Actions
Ovaries	
Estrogen	Stimulates development and maintenance of secondary sex characteristics Stimulates protein anabolism Prepares endometrium for implantation of fertilized ovum
Progesterone	Prepares uterus for pregnancy Prepares breasts for lactation Promotes protein catabolism
Testes	
Testosterone	Stimulates ▼ Development and maintenance of primary and secondary sex characteristics in boys ▼ Sperm production ▼ Protein anabolism for growth

Modified from Wong, D: *Whaley and Wong's nursing care of infants and children,* ed 5, St Louis, 1995, Mosby.

Table 9-2. Summary of Pediatric Endocrine Diagnostic Tests

Procedure	Purpose	Indications
Bone-age radiographic test	Comparison of hand or wrist radiograph to standards for age	Hypothyroidism Growth hormone deficiency Precocious puberty—abnormally early onset of puberty Hyperthyroidism
Stimulation tests		
Growth hormone stimulation	Diagnose growth hormone deficiency	Growth hormone deficiency
Thyroid releasing hormone	Diagnose thyroid disease	Hypothyroidism Hyperthyroidism
Glucose tolerance	Assess glucose tolerance	Acromegaly
Provactive blood testing	Evaluate function of endocrine system by specific growth hormones	Growth hormone deficiency Adrenal insufficiency

Table 9-3. Commonly Used Medications for Endocrine Dysfunction

Classification	Medication	Indication	Route and Dosage	Side Effects	Nursing Implications
Hormone, thyroid	Generic: levothyrodine sodium Trade: Synthroid	Hypo-thyroidism	PO *6 to 12 months:* 50-75 mcg/day *1 to 5 years:* 75-100 mcg/day *6 to 12 years:* 100-150 mcg/day *>12 years:* 150 mcg/day IM, IV ½ to ¾ child's normal dosage	*CNS:* Nervousness, headache *CV:* Palpitations, tachycardia *Respiratory:* Shortness of breath *GI:* Change in appetite, vomiting *Integumentary:* Rash, hives *MS:* Muscle aches *Other:* Fever, heat sensitivity	Monitor BP and pulse Assess TSH, T_4, and T_3 Administer on empty stomach May crush tablet and mix with small amount of food *Parent education:* Administer medication at same time daily Do not administer with other OTC medications without physician approval Obtain follow-up to monitor thyroid levels Do not stop medication abruptly

Continued.

323

Table 9-3.   Commonly Used Medications for Endocrine Dysfunction—cont'd

Classification	Medication	Indication	Route and Dosage	Side Effects	Nursing Implications
Antidiabetic, hypoglycemic	Generic: regular, insulin zinc suspension prompt, regular human Trade: Regular, Semilente, Humulin-R, Novulin-R	Juvenile-onset diabetes (all types) Rapid acting	Individualized for child SC (DKA) (regular) 0.25-2 U/kg dose q 4-6 hrs IM, IV 0.1 U/kg bolus then 0.1 U/kg/hr	*Integumentary:* Urticaria, wheals, or lipodystrophy *Endocrine:* Hypoglycemia: tachycardia, nervousness Somogyi effect: Rebound hypoglycemia; get 3 A.M. blood sugar Hyperglycemia: Drowsiness, fruit-like breath odor, polyuria	Assess for symptoms of hyperglycemia or hypoglycemia When mixing, prepare clear (reg) to cloudy (NPH) Perform blood glucose monitoring as ordered *Parent and child education:* One nurse should coordinate teaching Assess readiness for learning Teach parents and child, if old enough, proper administration of insulin
	Generic: isophane insulin suspension Trade: NPH Generic: insulin zinc suspension Trade: Lente	Intermediate acting	Maintenance (Lente or NPH) 0.5 U/kg early A.M.		

Antidiabetic hypo- glycemic —cont'd	Intermediate acting	Generic: isophane human insulin suspension Trade: Novolin-N, Humulin-N	Site rotation, monitoring of side effects, importance of balanced diet, exercise, and rest Involve child in own care from beginning of treatment Have extra syringes and equipment on hand Discuss importance of ▶ hygiene ▶ footcare ▶ dental care ▶ eye examination ▶ medical-alert jewelry
		Long acting insulins are rarely used in children	

Table 9-4. Comparison of Manifestations: Hypoglycemia and Hyperglycemia

Variable	Hypoglycemia	Hyperglycemia
Onset	Rapid (minutes)	Gradual (days)
Mood	Labile, irritable, nervous, weepy	Lethargic
Mental status	Difficulty concentrating, speaking, focusing, coordinating	Dulled sensorium Confused
Inward feeling	Shakey feeling, hunger Headache Dizziness	Thirst Weakness Nausea/vomiting Abdominal pain
Skin	Pallor Sweating	Flushed Signs of dehydration
Mucous membranes	Normal	Dry, crusty
Respirations	Shallow, rapid	Deep, rapid (Kussmaul)
Pulse	Tachycardia	Less rapid, weak
Breath odor	Normal	Fruity, acetone
Neurologic	Tremors Late: hyperreflexia, dilated pupils, convulsion	Diminished reflexes Paresthesia
Ominous signs	Shock, coma	Acidosis, coma
Blood:		
Glucose	Low: below 60 mg/dl	High: 250 mg/dl or higher
Ketones	Negative/trace	High/large
Osmolarity	Normal	High from hemoconcentration
pH	Normal	Low (7.25 or less)
Hematocrit	Normal	High from hemoconcentration
HCO_3	Normal	Less than 20 mEq/L
Urine:		
Output	Normal	Polyuria (early) to oliguria (late)
Sugar	Negative	High
Acetone	Negative/trace	High

From Wong D: *Whaley and Wong's nursing care of infants and children,* ed 5, St Louis, 1995, Mosby.

REVIEW QUESTIONS

1. A 7-year-old child complains of shakiness, hunger, and headache. Based on these findings, the school nurse should suspect the student has which of these conditions?
   a. Diabetic ketoacidosis
   b. Hyperglycemia
   c. Hypoglycemia
   d. Polyphagia

2. An infant diagnosed with hypothyroidism has been ordered to receive levothyroxine (Synthroid) orally. The infant should be observed for signs of overdosage of this medication, which include
   a. Enuresis, dilated pupils, bradycardia
   b. Irritability, tachycardia, increased appetite
   c. Decreased blood pressure, intolerance to cold, tachycardia
   d. Bradycardia, constipation, tachypnea

3. If a child must receive daily insulin injections, which of these instructions should be given?
   a. Insulin is injected at a 90 degree angle while holding the skin tightly
   b. Needle length and gauge are unimportant in promoting comfort
   c. A rotation pattern for various parts of body will enhance absorption, since insulin has slowed absorption in overused areas
   d. Usual injection sites are thigh, hip, and periumbilical area

4. A mother of a newly diagnosed diabetic is receiving nutritional counseling. Which of these statements by the mother indicates the need for further teaching?
   a. "Calories and nutrient proportions have to be consistent on a daily basis"
   b. "Chocolate milk with meals is acceptable"
   c. "Meals and snacks must be eaten at the same time each day"
   d. "Cola may be exchanged for fruit juice"

5. The nurse is planning to teach the mother of an infant diagnosed with hypothyroidism about proper administration of levothyroxine (Synthroid). The teaching plan should include mixing the crushed medication in
   a. A 4 ounce bottle of formula
   b. Cherry syrup
   c. A small amount of baby food
   d. Fruit juice

6. Considering a 7-year-old child's diagnosis of ketoacidosis, the child is likely to exhibit which of the following symptoms?
   a. Frequent episodes of vomiting
   b. Dilated pupils
   c. Rapid, deep respirations
   d. Warm skin and diaphoresis

7. Which of these laboratory findings of an infant diagnosed with hypothyroidism is useful in determining whether the treatment is effective?
   a. Iodine level
   b. Tapazole level
   c. CPK, LDH, CK-MB
   d. Serum T_4 and T_3, TSH

8. The mother of a newly diagnosed diabetic asks why insulin needs to be injected. The nurse responds that the child cannot take oral insulin because it
   a. Is not tolerated well in oral form by children
   b. Is not available in pill form
   c. Is destroyed by digestive enzymes
   d. Will cause gastric ulcers

9. A school-age child with a diagnosis of juvenile diabetes has been taught the importance of site rotation for insulin administration. Which of these statements made by the child indicates a need for further teaching?
   a. "I won't use a site that contains bulges"
   b. "Once I find a comfortable site, I'll use it frequently"
   c. "I must record site of insulin injections"
   d. "I may use the abdomen, thighs, and arms as injection sites"

10. An infant has been diagnosed with hypothyroidism. Which one of the following nursing diagnoses should receive priority in the nursing care?
    a. Altered nutrition: less than body requirements
    b. Risk for impaired skin integrity
    c. Knowledge deficit
    d. Pain

ANSWERS, RATIONALES, AND TEST-TAKING TIPS

Rationales	Test-Taking Tips

1. **Correct answer: c**

Signs of hypoglycemia are caused by increased adrenergic activity and increased secretion of catecholamines, which produces nervousness, headaches, and hunger. Findings associated with diabetic ketoacidosis include dehydration from the diuresis; rapid, deep respirations; electrolyte imbalance; and metabolic acidosis. Findings associated with hyperglycemia include lethargy, deep and rapid respirations, and fruity, acetone breath. In option *d*, this is one of the three cardinal signs of diabetes (the "polys": polyphagia, polydipsia, and polyuria).

Relate the findings in the stem to an experience such as working all day without eating. You were probably shaky, hungry, and may have had a headache or become ill-tempered.

2. **Correct answer: b**

Most adverse reactions to thyroid agents result from toxicity and include irritability, tachycardia, and increased appetite. The heart rate and BP are increased.

The key word in the question is "overdosage." With too much thyroid, think of a hypermetabolic state in which all systems are strained to increase speed. To easily select the correct response, approach the responses by reading vertically the first series of items: enuresis—doesn't occur; irritability—does occur; decreased BP—doesn't occur; and bradycardia—doesn't occur. Next, read all the responses in *b* to ensure they are correct, which they are.

3. **Correct answer: c**

The child and parent are assisted by the nurse to create an appropriate rotation schedule. Insulin is injected at a 45 or 90 degree angle, which is altered according to the thickness of the layer of adipose tissue at a specific site. The smallest needle length and gauge that delivers insulin to the subcutaneous tissue should be chosen. Typically, a 25 or 27 gauge and ⅝ inch needle are used. Absorption has been demonstrated to be more rapid in the arms, less rapid in the abdomen, and slowest in the thigh.

An approach to these responses is to cluster a, b, and d as specific data. Response c is more complete, comprehensive, and the best selection.

4. **Correct answer: b**

Low-carbohydrate snacks are emphasized in the diabetic's diet. Nutritional counseling emphasizes a constant menu and complex carbohydrates. Consistent meal times are emphasized. Substitutions with foods of equal carbohydrate content are usually acceptable without affecting the blood glucose control.

The most important approach to use with these type of questions is careful reading. Be sure to note "the need for further reading." Select an incorrect statement, option b. Before moving to the next question simply reread the question once more and then read your response to ensure you have chosen the best option.

5. **Correct answer: c**

For infants, crushed medications should be mixed with 1 teaspoon of a sweet food such as applesauce. Medication should not be mixed in

Cluster the two responses that do not include amounts, options b and d. Of the remaining options select the smallest volume, which is option c.

formula. Flavored syrup, in a small amount, is an acceptable medium in which to mix crushed medication. However, this option does not include the amount of syrup to be used. Medications should not be mixed in essential food items, since the child may later refuse them.

6. Correct answer: c

In this metabolic acidotic state, the respiratory system attempts to return the pH to normal by eliminating the CO_2 through an increase in the depth and rate of respirations described as Kussmaul's respirations. Nausea and vomiting are early findings consistent with hyperglycemia before the client is in ketoacidosis. The findings in options *b* and *d* are consistent with hypoglycemia.

Remember *K*etoacidosis is associated with *K*ussmaul's. Note that in both hyperglycemia and hypoglycemia the respiratory rate is rapid; the difference is that in hyperglycemia breathing is deep and in hypoglycemia, shallow.

7. Correct answer: d

Effective treatment is determined by a restoration of the state of euthyroid—normal T_3, T_4, and TSH. Iodine is essential for thyroid hormone production. Tapazole is prescribed for hyperthyroidism. The items in response *c* are cardiac enzymes used for the detection of myocardial damage when they elevate.

Remember the three *T*s (serum tests for *T*hyroid function): T_3, T_4, and TSH (thyroid stimulating hormone from the anterior pituitary).

8. **Correct answer: c**

Insulin is not effective when taken orally because the GI tract breaks down the protein molecule before it can be absorbed and reach the bloodstream. Type 1 diabetes mellitus, typically found in children, requires exogenous insulin to control the blood glucose level, since the pancreas, Beta cells, does not produce any insulin. Oral hypoglycemic agents that are available in oral form are given to patients with type II diabetes, which is usually diagnosed in middle age. This type results when the pancreas does not produce enough insulin; the oral hypoglycemics stimulate the pancreas to produce more insulin. Option *d* is a false statement.

Eliminate initially that which you know is false, option *d*. Eliminate option *a* since it is unlikely that all children wouldn't tolerate a medication. Next make an educated guess that if option *c* happened, then option *b* would follow. Thus, select option *c,* which best answers the question.

9. **Correct answer: b**

Lipoatrophy, a breakdown of subcutaneous fat, occurs after several injections at the same site. Lipohypertrophy is the buildup of subcutaneous fat tissue at the site of an insulin injection. Insulin lipodystrophy is the loss of local fat deposits in diabetic clients as a complication of repeated insulin injections. Options *a, c,* and *d* are correct statements that

The use of common sense will facilitate the selection of the correct answer: with injection of any substance, the same site should not be used repeatedly.

indicate the child needs no further education. Children should avoid sites with lipohypertrophy. Recording the sites of insulin injection is emphasized to prevent overutilization of any one site; all listed sites are appropriate for self-injection of insulin.

10. Correct answer: a

A major finding of hypothyroidism is slow growth and metabolism from thyroid hormone deprivation. Thyroid hormones are responsible for many diverse effects including growth and development, normal function of the bowel, and regulation of metabolic rate and protein synthesis. Option *c* is an appropriate nursing diagnosis related to family education in thyroxine therapy. Option *a*, altered nutrition, will be resolved once thyroid hormone is given to the infant. Option *b* is not an appropriate nursing diagnosis for thyroid dysfunction. Option *d* is not a usual finding of hyperthyroidism or hypothyroidism.

Use Maslow's hierarchy of needs after you have narrowed the responses to either *a* or *c*, since options *b* and *d* have no information in the stem to support their selection. Select option *c* since physiologic needs are priorities and the client is an infant. The family needs knowledge about medication administration in order to deal with the improvement of nutrition, option *a*.

Nursing Care of Children with Special Needs

STUDY OUTCOMES

After completing this chapter, the reader will be able to do the following:

▼ Identify strategies for assisting families with a child who has special needs.

▼ Describe nursing interventions to be used when interacting with a child who has a sensory impairment.

▼ List general classifications of hearing impairment.

▼ Identify major classifications of mental retardation.

▼ Describe nursing interventions appropriate when caring for a cognitively impaired child.

▼ Outline a plan of care for a child with a severe burn.

KEY TERMS

Amblyopia	Reduced vision in an eye that appears to be structurally normal when examined by an ophthalmoscope; such condition may lead to strabismus.
Conductive hearing loss	Form of hearing loss in which sound is inadequately conducted through the external or middle ear to the sensorineural apparatus of the inner ear; sensitivity to sound is diminished, but clarity (interpretation of sound) is not changed.
Corium	Also called the **dermis**. A layer of skin, just below the epidermis, consisting of papillary and reticular layers and containing blood and lymphatic vessels, nerves, nerve endings, glands and hair follicles.
Curling ulcer	Also called **curlings stress ulcer**. A duodenal ulcer that develops in people who have severe burns on the surface of the body.
Epithelium	Covering of the internal and external organs of the body, lining of vessels, body cavities, glands, and organs; the cells are bound together by connective tissue.
Hydrotherapy	Use of water in the treatment of various physical or mental disorders.
Hyperopia	Also called **hypermetropia, hypermetropy.** Farsightedness, a condition resulting from an error of refraction in which rays of light entering the eye are brought into focus behind the retina.
Myopia	Also called **short sight.** Condition of nearsightedness caused by the elongation of the eyeball or by an error in refraction so that parallel rays are focused in front of the retina.
Porcine xenograft	Also called **heterograft**. A temporary biological graft from the skin of a pig used to cover a burn during the first few days, reducing the amount of fluid loss from the open wound; this type of graft is rejected quickly.
Rinne test	Also called **rinne tuning fork test.** A method of distinguishing conductive from sensorineural hearing loss; sensorineural loss—sound heard longer by air conduction; conductive loss—sound heard longer by bone conduction.

Sensorineural hearing loss	Form of hearing loss in which sound is conducted normally through the external and middle ear, but a defect in the inner ear or auditory nerve results in hearing loss; sound discrimination may or may not be affected.
Snellen chart	Chart used in testing visual acuity by letters, numbers or symbols arranged on the chart in decreasing size from top to bottom; the test is done from a distance of 20 feet.
Strabismus	Abnormal ocular condition in which the eyes are crossed.
Weber test	Method of assessment in auditory acuity, especially useful in determining whether defective hearing in an ear is a conductive loss caused by middle ear problems or a sensorineural loss; a vibrating tuning fork is placed in the center of the person's forehead, the midline vertex, or the maxillary incisor; if there is sensorineural loss in one ear, the unaffected ear perceives the sound as louder; if conductive hearing loss is present, the sound is louder in the affected ear, because sound is received only by bone conduction.

CONTENT REVIEW

I. **Attention deficit–hyperactivity disorder (AD–HD)**
   A. Description: syndrome of varying severity characterized by learning and behavior disabilities; affects children, adolescents, and, rarely, adults
   B. Etiology and incidence
      1. Frequency is 10 times more common in males than in females
      2. Exact cause is unknown; brain illness or trauma before, during, or after birth is likely involved
      3. Other factors involved include neurotransmitter abnormality, maturational lag; hypersensitivity to food items or additives is controversial
   C. Assessment
      1. Assessment findings: (Box 10-1, p. 352)
      2. Diagnostic evaluation
         a. Complete medical and developmental history

      b. Home and school observation of behavior

      c. Physical examination, including detailed neurologic workup

      d. Psychologic testing to determine intelligence and achievement levels, visual-perceptual difficulties

      e. Screen for other potential causes: lead poisoning, hearing loss, seizures

D. Therapeutic management

    1. Behavioral therapy and psychotherapy—behavior modification techniques, family counseling

    2. Medication: stimulants, sympathomimetic amines—methylphenidate (Ritalin)—to reduce symptoms of the disorder

    3. Diet—controversial

    4. Appropriate classroom placement—small, orderly, structured setting with minimal distractions and stimuli

E. Nursing management: acute/home care

    1. Nursing diagnosis: risk for injury

    2. Expected outcome: the child participates in a structured environment in school

    3. Interventions

      a. Assess child's environment for safety hazards

      b. Recommend elimination of excess sugar, if child has demonstrated sensitivity

      c. Administer stimulant as ordered

      d. Teach parents correct administration of stimulant; explain side effects

    4. Nursing diagnosis: compromised ineffective family coping

    5. Expected outcome: the child and family discuss/implement effective coping strategies

    6. Interventions

      a. Assess coping strategies currently being used by family and child

      b. Refer child for individual psychotherapy in addition to family therapy

      c. Review effective parenting techniques, including discipline and rewarding for appropriate behavior

    7. Additional nursing diagnoses

      a. Self-esteem disturbance

      b. Impaired social interaction

      c. Caregiver role strain

F. **Evaluation**
  1. Parents demonstrate correct administration of stimulant
  2. Parents demonstrate effective parenting techniques
  3. Child and family demonstrate effective coping strategies
  4. Child functions within expected limits in school environment

II. Mental retardation (MR)

A. **Description: disorder characterized by below average general intellectual function (IQ of 70 or below); classifications include mild, moderate, severe, and profound levels of deficit**
B. **Etiology and incidence**
  1. Causes
     a. Severe—genetic, biochemical, infectious, developmental
     b. Mild—maternal lifestyle factors: cigarette smoking, poor nutrition, and chemical abuse
  2. Down syndrome accounts for 25% of all cases of MR
C. **Assessment**
  1. Psychometric testing: Stanford-Binet, Wechsler Intelligence Scale for Children (Revised) to determine level of disability and function
  2. Behaviors
     a. Delayed developmental milestones
     b. Poor eye contact during feeding
     c. Nonresponsiveness
     d. Irritability
     e. Decreased spontaneous activity
  3. Family assessment
D. **Therapeutic management**
  1. Infant stimulation program
  2. Skills: ADLs, self-help, verbal, social, and adaptive behaviors
  3. Behavior modification
E. **Nursing management**
  1. Nursing diagnosis: altered growth and development
  2. Expected outcomes
     a. Child and family participate in infant stimulation program
     b. Child's maximal potential for development is realized
  3. Interventions
     a. Review recent psychological and physical assessment findings; assess child's current level of functioning
     b. Involve family in early intervention programs: infant stimulation

      c. Assist family in setting realistic goals for child

      d. Encourage learning of self-care skills

      e. Assist family in locating special daycare programs and educational classes, including vocational training

      f. Emphasize need for limit-setting, discipline, social interaction, preparation for sexual maturation

   4. Nursing diagnosis: altered family processes

   5. Expected outcome: family demonstrates acceptance of child

   6. Interventions

      a. Assist family with decision to care for child at home or locate residential site for placement

      b. Emphasize child's strengths and potential abilities

      c. Encourage verbalization of concerns and feelings related to the child

      d. Provide information regarding support services, community agencies, and opportunities for socialization

   7. Additional nursing diagnoses

      a. Knowledge deficit

      b. Anxiety

F. Evaluation

   1. Family demonstrates acceptance of child

   2. Child and family participate in support services

III. Sensory impairment

A. Description: those impairments leading to visual and/or auditory deprivation that place children at risk for impaired cognitive, perceptive, communication, and socialization development skills

B. Etiology and incidence

   1. Common visual disorders in childhood include refractive disorders (myopia, hyperopia), strabismus, injury from foreign bodies, and conjunctivitis

   2. Auditory disturbances are classified as conductive, sensorineural, or mixed type

   3. Damage to inner structures or auditory nerve, infection, ototoxic drugs, excessive exposure to loud noises cause sensorineural hearing loss

   4. Conductive hearing loss is caused by middle ear infection

C. Assessment

   1. Assessment findings

      a. Visual: symptoms depend on type of visual impairment (Table 10-1, pp. 353-355)

    b. Auditory
        (1) Infant
            (a) Lack of startle or blink reflex to loud sound
            (b) Failure to localize sounds by 6 months of age
            (c) Absence of babble or vocalization by 7 months of age
        (2) Child
            (a) Failure to develop intelligible speech by 2 years of age
            (b) Use of gestures to indicate desires rather than verbalization after 15 months of age
            (c) Vocal play, head banging, or foot stamping for vibratory sensation

2. Diagnostic studies: early discovery of sensory problems is essential
    a. Vision
        (1) Snellen test: E symbol or letter (for children able to read alphabet) to determine distant visual acuity
        (2) Cover-uncover test to determine eye muscle imbalance
    b. Hearing
        (1) Audiometry to determine degree of hearing loss
        (2) Rinne and Weber tests
        (3) Tympanometry reveals middle ear pressure

D. **Therapeutic management**
    1. Medications
        a. Antibiotics—opthalamic ointments to treat eye infection; oral antibiotics to treat middle ear infection
        b. Antiinflammatories—to decrease eye inflammation
    2. Surgery
        a. Vision: corrective surgery for strabismus and eye trauma
        b. Hearing: cochlear implants for sensorineural loss; insertion of tympanotomy tubes for otitis media
    3. Other treatments
        a. Vision: corrective lens, patching
        b. Hearing: hearing aids, speech therapy, sign language, use of telecommunication device

E. **Nursing management for the hospitalized child with a sensory deficit: nursing diagnoses with interventions**
    1. Vision
        a. Sensory perceptual alteration: visual

    b. Expected outcome: child demonstrates progression in developmental tasks

    c. Interventions

        (1) Assess visual acuity; perform or facilitate visual tests for acuity, strabismus, and amblyopia as indicated

        (2) Face child when speaking; offer explanation of what is happening in the environment

        (3) Orient child to room; arrange furniture with child's safety in mind

        (4) State name when entering room; explain any procedure before starting

        (5) Assist with correct use of corrective devices

        (6) Administer opthalamic medications as ordered

        (7) Teach family correct method of administering medications

        (8) Provide information regarding special programs to learn independent behavior, braille reading and writing

        (9) Provide toys that stimulate the senses of hearing and touch

2. Hearing

    a. Sensory-perceptual alteration: auditory

    b. Expected outcome: child adapts to hearing loss and maintains independence in activities

    c. Interventions

        (1) Assess auditory acuity

        (2) Facilitate auditory testing to determine degree of hearing loss

        (3) Face child when speaking and speak slowly and distinctly, without shouting

        (4) Assist with use of a hearing aid

        (5) Teach family proper use and care of a hearing device

        (6) Provide family with information regarding rehabilitation programs; encourage the learning of sign language

        (7) Instruct parents to provide stimulation through language

        (8) Provide information on amplification devices for phone, teletypewriters, signaling devices for doorbell, and phone and closed-captioned television

(9) Assist parents to select toys that promote social interaction and increase potential for hearing
3. Additional nursing diagnoses
   a. Altered growth and development
   b. Risk for injury
   c. Altered family processes
F. Evaluation
   1. Child maintains independence with progression in developmental tasks
   2. Child correctly uses assistive devices or aids
   3. Family participates in formal rehabilitation program or support services

IV. Burns
A. Etiology and incidence
   1. Second leading cause of death from trauma in childhood
   2. Most likely age group requiring hospitalization as a result of burns are children less than 4 years of age
   3. Causes of burns
      a. Thermal agents—flame, direct contact, hot water, steam
      b. Chemical agents—acids or alkali
      c. Electrical agents—electrical cords
      d. Radioactive agents—x-rays or ultraviolet exposure
   4. House fires cause the majority of fire fatalities; the majority of burn injuries are caused by thermal agents
B. Pathophysiology
   1. Extent of tissue destruction is related to heat source intensity, duration of contact, and speed by which heat energy is dissipated by burned surface
   2. There are standardized charts to estimate distribution of burns in children less than 5 years and older children (Figure 10-1); expressed as percentage of total body surface area. Note: the standard "rule of nines" used for adults is not appropriate for young children.
   3. Current classification of burn depth of tissue injury
      a. Superficial (first degree)—minimal tissue damage, painful
      b. Partial thickness burn (second degree)—involves epithelium and portion of corium, very painful
      c. Full thickness burn (third and fourth degree)—skin of all layers destroyed, as well as underlying tissues, no pain

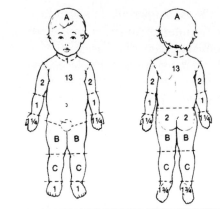

RELATIVE PERCENTAGES OF AREAS AFFECTED BY GROWTH

AREA	BIRTH	AGE 1 YR	AGE 5 YR
A = ½ of head	9½	8½	6½
B = ½ of one thigh	2¾	3¼	4
C = ½ of one leg	2½	2½	2¾

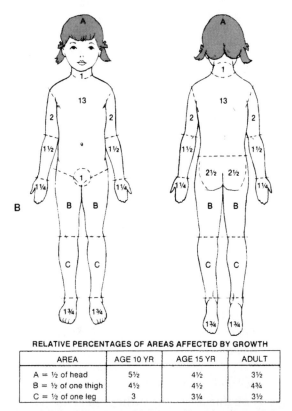

RELATIVE PERCENTAGES OF AREAS AFFECTED BY GROWTH

AREA	AGE 10 YR	AGE 15 YR	ADULT
A = ½ of head	5½	4½	3½
B = ½ of one thigh	4½	4½	4¾
C = ½ of one leg	3	3¼	3½

Figure 10-1. Extent of burn injury. **A,** Children from birth to age 5 years; **B,** Older children. (From Wong, D: *Whaley and Wong's nursing care of infants and children,* ed 5, St Louis, 1995, Mosby.)

4. Burns are assessed according to severity
   a. Minor burns: partial thickness burns of <10% total body surface area in children; full-thickness burns of <2% of BSA offer no risk of cosmetic or functional impairment or disability
   b. Moderate burns: partial thickness burns of 10% to 25% total body surface area; full thickness burns of <10% of BSA; offer minimal risk of cosmetic or functional impairment except in small children or when the burns involve critical areas such as the face, feet, hands, or genitalia in children <10 years of age
   c. Major or critical burns: partial-thickness burns of 25% total BSA in children; full-thickness burns of 10% of BSA or more; burns involving the face, eyes, ears, hands, feet, and perineum; high-voltage electric burn injury; all burn injuries associated with chemical, inhalation, or major trauma; major burns are likely to result in functional or cosmetic impairment or disability
   d. Burns of the face, hands, feet, or perineum, even though small in area, often require hospitalization as a result of the risk of airway obstruction, severe hypoxia, and rapid fluid shifts
5. Local and systemic responses of the body to an initial burn injury
   a. Local
      (1) Edema formation—results from altered hydrostatic pressure and capillary permeability
      (2) Fluid and protein loss—as a result of skin loss
      (3) Reduced blood flow to affected area
   b. Systemic
      (1) Burn shock—from reduced circulation which results in a decreased cardiac output
      (2) Acidosis
      (3) Reduced renal perfusion
      (4) Increased metabolic rate and altered growth rate
6. Three phases of burn care
   a. Emergent: begins immediately after the injury as the body reacts with an inflammatory response and a large shift of extracellular fluid in to the damaged tissues
      (1) Usually lasts 2 days
      (2) Priorities include
         (a) Assess the ABCs (airway, breathing, and circulation)
         (b) Assess for associated trauma
         (c) Conserve body heat—cover nonburned areas

        (d) Administer fluids—a priority at this time to prevent shock

        (e) Monitor serum potassium levels, which are typically elevated

  b. Acute: occurs during the time wound is healing until wound closure

    (1) Begins on day 3 and lasts to about 3 months

    (2) Priorities

        (a) Monitor for fluid overload

        (b) Prevent infection

        (c) Wound care

        (d) Nutritional support

        (e) Pain management

        (f) Physical therapy

  c. Rehabilitation: occurs as the child attempts to return to an optimal level of function;

    (1) May last a few years up to a lifetime

    (2) Priorities

        (a) Regaining of independence

        (b) Prevention or minimization of deformities and scarring

        (c) Contracture or scar revisions

        (d) Emotional support

        (e) Physical and occupational therapy

7. Burn complications in children

  a. Inhalation injury to upper and lower airways

  b. Acute bronchitis and bronchopneumonia

  c. Wound sepsis

  d. Curling or stress ulcer

  e. CNS dysfunction: including hallucinations, seizures, and coma

  f. Arterial hypertension

C. Assessment

  1. Wound condition

  2. Child's overall condition and behaviors

  3. Signs of complications

  4. Need for pain management if first or second degree burns are present

D. Therapeutic management

  1. Debridement in conjunction with hydrotherapy

  2. Methods of burn wound covering

    a. Exposure—wounds left open to air

        b. Open wound left uncovered with antimicrobial cream or ointment applied

        c. Modified—cream or ointment applied directly to wound or by means of thin gauze; wound then covered with gauze or net covering

        d. Occlusive—cream-impregnated gauze placed on wound, layers of bulky gauze applied, secured with stretched gauze or net

   3. Topical antimicrobials most commonly used

        a. 1% silver sulfadiazine (Silvadene): causes a sensation of coldness when applied; effective against many gram-positive and gram-negative organisms; allergic reaction—burning, stinging, swelling

        b. 10% mafenide acetate (Sulfamylon): causes discomfort when applied; effective against many gram-positive and gram-negative organisms; effective in deep flame and eclectic wounds

        c. 0.5% silver nitrate solution: stains skin, linens, and clothes; effective against Pseudomonas and staphlycoccus; does not interfere with wound healing; difficult to apply

   4. Skin grafts

        a. Temporary grafts include homografts and heterografts; porcine (pigskin) xenograft commonly used in children

        b. Permanent grafts include autografts and isografts

E. Nursing management

   1. Nursing diagnoses with interventions

        a. Emergent phase

           (1) Nursing diagnosis: impaired gas exchange

           (2) Expected outcome: child demonstrates improved gas exchange, as manifested by respirations between 16 and 24 (child), and clear bilateral breath sounds

           (3) Interventions

               (a) Assess for signs of respiratory distress: restlessness, confusion, labored breathing, diminished or adventitious breath sounds

               (b) Monitor ABCs as ordered

               (c) Continuously monitor SaO_2 levels

               (d) Administer O_2 as ordered

               (e) Elevate the head of the bed

           (4) Nursing diagnosis: risk for fluid volume deficit

           (5) Expected outcome: fluid volume is restored with appropriate potassium levels

    (6) Interventions
        (a) Assess for signs of fluid volume deficit
        (b) Monitor vital signs
        (c) Monitor potassium levels and urine for specific gravity
        (d) Monitor I&O and hourly urine output
        (e) Assess daily weights
        (f) Monitor Hgb and Hct
        (g) Observe for signs of curling ulcer or hemorrhage: bloody or coffee-brown emesis, melena, epigastric pain, or abdominal distention
        (h) Administer IV fluids and electrolytes as ordered
        (i) Administer diuretic and albumin as ordered
        (j) Administer antacids or H_2-histamine receptor antagonists to decrease risk of gastric bleeding

b. Emergent and acute phase
    (1) Nursing diagnoses
        (a) Impaired skin integrity
        (b) Risk for infection
    (2) Expected outcome: child maintains skin integrity without infection
    (3) Interventions
        (a) Assess percentage of body surface burned, using appropriate chart (emergent)
        (b) Assess burn condition and location (emergent)
        (c) Assess level of pain (emergent and acute)
        (d) Assess for signs of infection: drainage, odor, delayed healing, change in vital signs
        (e) Maintain infection control techniques
        (f) Enforce strict hand washing
        (g) Use hydrotherapy tub, as ordered, to cleanse and debride
        (h) Apply bacteriostatic agent as ordered
        (i) Maintain extremities in alignment to prevent contractures
        (j) Dress wounds as ordered
        (k) D through j are interventions for acute phase
    (4) Nursing diagnosis: altered nutrition—less than body requirements
    (5) Expected outcome: child has adequate nutrition, as evidenced by maintenance of 90% of preburn weight

    (6) Interventions
     (a) Obtain child's weight before injury
     (b) Assess eating habits, preferred foods, food allergies
     (c) Maintain calorie count
     (d) Assess daily weights
     (e) Provide high-calorie, high-protein diet, supplemented with high doses of vitamins B, C, iron, and zinc
     (f) Gradually increase liquid diet to regular diet
     (g) Encourage family to bring favorite foods from home
     (h) Provide nutritious between-meal snacks
     (i) Provide positive reinforcement for eating
  c. Rehabilitation phase
    (1) Nursing diagnosis: body image disturbance
    (2) Expected outcome: child exhibits behaviors that indicate body image has been restored or maintained
    (3) Interventions
     (a) Assess child for feelings related to the change in appearance, difficulty with school and social situations; monitor for withdrawal or depression
     (b) Encourage child to express feelings and concerns related to restrictions in lifestyle, altered appearance
     (c) Support child in decision making
     (d) Discuss with family the impact of the burns on body systems
     (e) Stress importance of family support and child participation in peer activities
     (f) Suggest follow-up counseling with child-life worker or counselor
 2. Other nursing diagnoses
  a. Emergent phase
    (1) Pain
    (2) Risk for injury: paralytic ileus
    (3) Ineffective airway clearance
    (4) Impaired physical mobility
  b. Acute phase
    (1) Risk for fluid overload
    (2) Risk for altered tissue perfusion
    (3) Risk for altered nutrition: less than body requirements
    (4) Anxiety/fear

        c. Rehabilitation phase
           (1) Ineffective family processes
           (2) Self-care deficit

  F. **Evaluation**
     1. Child exhibits an absence of fluid and electrolyte imbalance
     2. Child exhibits an absence of skin impairment and infection
     3. Child verbalizes improved body image and makes social contacts outside of the family
     4. Family seeks psychological counseling as necessary

V. The abused child

  A. **Description: the physical or psychological assault or neglect of a child**
  B. **Etiology and incidence**
     1. More than 2 million children receive protective services each year
     2. Three factors predispose child to physical injury by parents or other caregivers
        a. Parental characteristics—parents have been victims themselves
        b. Child characteristics—temperament, physical or cognitive disability predispose child to injury, illegitimacy, or hyperactivity
        c. Environmental characteristics—divorce, marital problems, financial strain, alcoholism, drug addiction, poor housing
  C. **Assessment (Table 10-2, p. 356)**
  D. **Nursing management**
     1. Nursing diagnoses with interventions
        a. Nursing diagnosis: risk for injury
        b. Expected outcome: child is free of additional abuse
        c. Interventions
           (1) Assess child for injury, fractures, burns
           (2) Assess interpersonal relationship between child and family
           (3) Assess child's reaction to healthcare personnel
           (4) Assess history or present evidence of injury
           (5) Complete thorough history in nonthreatening manner
           (6) Provide safe environment for child
           (7) Provide treatment for current injury
           (8) Document thoroughly: child's physical condition, child's interaction with parents, interview with family
           (9) Report findings to proper authorities
          (10) Establish a therapeutic relationship with family

        d. Nursing diagnoses
            (1) Fear/anxiety
            (2) Altered parenting
        e. Expected outcome: family exhibits positive interaction with child
        f. Interventions
            (1) Assess current support systems
            (2) Provide consistent caregiver to enhance trust and consistency
            (3) Provide care for child until parent is ready to participate
            (4) Provide parent opportunity to verbalize emotions
            (5) Participate in multidisciplinary approach
            (6) Refer parents to special support groups and counseling
            (7) Teach parents regarding effective child-rearing techniques, child growth and development
    2. Additional nursing diagnoses
        a. Knowledge deficit
        b. Self-concept disturbance
        c. Altered skin integrity
        d. Altered family processes

3. Evaluation

    1. Child is free from additional injury
    2. Parents demonstrate appropriate parenting activities
    3. Parents participate in counseling and support services

Box 10-1. Diagnostic Criteria for Attention Deficit–Hyperactivity Disorder

Note: Consider a criterion met only if the behavior is considerably more frequent than that of most people of the same mental age.

A. A disturbance of at least 6 months during which at least eight of the following are present:

    (1) Often fidgets with hands or feet or squirms in seat (in adolescents, may be limited to subjective feelings of restlessness)

    (2) Has difficulty remaining seated when required to do so

    (3) Is easily distracted by extraneous stimuli

    (4) Has difficulty awaiting turn in games or group situations

    (5) Often blurts out answers to questions before they have been completed

    (6) Has difficulty following through on instructions from others (not due to oppositional behavior or failure of comprehension), e.g., fails to finish chores

    (7) Has difficulty sustaining attention in tasks or play activities

    (8) Often shifts from one uncompleted activity to another

    (9) Has difficulty playing quietly

    (10) Often talks excessively

    (11) Often interrupts or intrudes on others, e.g., butts into other children's games

    (12) Often does not seem to listen to what is being said to him or her

    (13) Often loses things necessary for tasks or activities at school or at home (e.g., toys, pencils, books, assignments)

    (14) Often engages in physically dangerous activities without considering possible consequences (not for the purpose of thrill-seeking) e.g., runs into street without looking

Note: The above items are listed in descending order of discriminating power based on data from a national field trial of the DSM-III-R criteria for Disruptive Behavior Disorders.

B. Onset before the age of seven

C. Does not meet the criteria for a Pervasive Developmental Disorder

Criteria for Severity of Attention Deficit–Hyperactivity Disorder:

Mild: Few, if any symptoms in excess of those required to make the diagnosis and only minimal or no impairment in school and social functioning

Moderate: Symptoms or functional impairment intermediate between "mild" and "severe"

Severe: Many symptoms in excess of those required to make the diagnosis and significant and pervasive impairment in functioning at home and school and with peers

From Diagnostic and statistical manual of mental disorders, ed 4—revised (DSM IV), Washington, DC, 1994, American Psychiatric Association.
In Wong, D: *Whaley and Wong's nursery care of infants and children,* ed 5, St Louis, 1995, Mosby.

Table 10-1. Types of Visual Impairment

Defect/Description	Pathophysiology	Clinical Manifestations	Treatment
Refractive errors			
Myopia (nearsightedness)—ability to see objects clearly at close range but not at a distance	Results from eyeball that is too long, causing image to fall in front of retina	*Behavioral manifestations:* Rubs eyes excessively Tilts head or thrusts head forward Has difficulty in reading or other close work Holds books close to eyes Writes or colors with head close to table Clumsy; walks into objects Blinks more than usual or is irritable when doing close work Is unable to see objects clearly Does poorly in school, especially in subjects that require demonstration such as arithmetic *Signs/symptoms:* Dizziness Headache Nausea following close work	Corrected with biconcave lenses that focus rays on retina

Continued.

Table 10-1. Types of Visual Impairment—cont'd

Defect/Description	Pathophysiology	Clinical Manifestations	Treatment
Refractive errors—cont'd			
Hyperopia (hypermetropia or farsightedness)—ability to see objects clearly at a distance but not at close range	Results from eyeball that is too short, causing image to focus beyond retina	Because of accommodative ability, child can usually see objects at all ranges Most children normally hyperopic until about 7 years of age	If correction is required, use convex lenses to focus rays on retina
Astigmatism—unequal curvatures in refractive apparatus	Results from unequal curvatures in cornea or lens that cause light rays to bend in different directions	Depends on severity of refractive error in each eye May have clinical manifestations of myopia	Corrected with special lenses that compensate for refractive errors
Anisometropia—different refractive strengths in each eye	May develop amblyopia as weaker eye is used less	Depends on severity of refractive error in each eye May have clinical manifestations of myopia Poor vision in affected eye	Treated with corrective lenses, preferably contact lenses, to improve vision in each eye so they work as a unit
Amblyopia ("lazy eye")—reduced visual acuity in one eye	Results when one eye does not receive sufficient stimulation Each retina receives different images, resulting in diplopia (double vision) Brain accommodates by suppressing less intense image Visual cortex eventually does not respond to visual stimulation with loss of vision in that eye		Preventable if treatment of primary visual defect such as anisometropia or strabismus begins before 6 years of age

Strabismus ("squint" or "cross-eye")—malalignment of eyes
Esotropia—inward deviation of eye
Extropia—outward deviation of eye

May result from muscle imbalance or paralysis, poor vision, or congenital defect
Since visual axes not parallel, brain receives two images, and amblyopia can result

Behavioral manifestations:
Squints eyelids together or frowns
Has difficulty in focusing from one distance to another
Inaccurate judgment in picking up objects
Unable to see print or moving objects clearly
Closes one eye to see
Tilts head to one side
If combined with refractive errors, may see any of the manifestations listed for refractive errors
Signs/symptoms:
Diplopia
Photophobia
Dizziness
Headache
Cross-eye

Treatment depends on cause of strabismus
May involve occlusion therapy (patching stronger eye) to increase visual stimulation to weaker eye
Early diagnosis essential to prevent vision loss

Modified from Wong, D: *Whaley and Wong's nursing care of infants and children*, ed 5, St Louis, 1995, Mosby.

Table 10-2. Assessment Findings of Various Forms of Abuse

Type of Abuse	Assessment Findings	Behavior Findings
Physical abuse	Bruises, welts Burns Fractures Lacerations and abrasions	Wary of adult physical contact Withdrawal Lack of reaction to frightening events Aggression
Physical neglect	Failure to thrive Malnutrition Poor personal hygiene Poor healthcare	Dull, apathetic Self-stimulating behavior Poor school attendance Drug or alcohol use
Sexual abuse	Bruises or lacerations on external genitalia Painful urination Difficulty sitting or walking Recurring UTI Venereal disease	Withdrawal Difficulty with peer relationships Sexual promiscuity Regressive behavior Rapidly declining school performance Fears and phobias
Emotional abuse	Failure to thrive Enuresis Sleep disorders Delayed physical development	Antisocial behavior, deteriorating conduct Suicide attempts Withdrawal Delayed emotional and cognitive development Increased anxiety, fears

From Wong, D: *Whaley and Wong's nursing care of infants and children,* ed 5, St Louis, 1995, Mosby.

REVIEW QUESTIONS

1. The nurse obtains all of the following data regarding an 18-month-old child suspected of being abused. Which comment by the mother should be reported?
   a. "I blame myself for this injury"
   b. "I want to know what is going to be done for my child"
   c. "I wish my child would be potty trained"
   d. "My sister helps care for my child"

2. A 7-year-old is diagnosed with attention deficit–hyperactivity disorder. To promote the child's optimal functioning, which of these approaches should be used?
   a. Encourage use of a delayed reward system
   b. Encourage a diet that emphasizes processed foods
   c. Obtain a placement in a structured, small classroom
   d. Obtain a prescription for antidepressant medications

3. A parent of a severely burned child has received information regarding the importance of nutritional support. Which of these diet selections made by the mother indicates an understanding of what she has been taught?
   a. Beef and cheese taco, yogurt, and skim milk
   b. Cheeseburger, celery and carrot sticks, cola
   c. Chicken nuggets, milkshake, and pudding
   d. Tossed salad, cheese sticks, banana, and tea

4. A school-age child, receiving methylphenidate (Ritalin), should be observed for the most common side effects, which are
   a. Nervousness and insomnia
   b. Heat sensitivity and polycythemia
   c. Signs of bleeding and bruising
   d. Vomiting and diarrhea

5. When a child is admitted to the hospital with suspected child abuse, the nurse is aware that legal proceedings may be necessary. Because of this possibility, which of these actions should receive priority?
   a. Assessing the child's developmental level
   b. Determining the extent of child's injuries
   c. Documenting physical findings and interactions during admission
   d. Informing parents about diagnostic tests

6. A preschooler is admitted to the hospital with moderate burns sustained in a house fire. He has sustained partial-thickness burns over 20% of his body surface area, including his hands and feet. Because of the client's condition, which of these nursing diagnoses should receive priority on admission to the hospital unit?
   a. Altered parenting
   b. Fluid volume deficit
   c. Knowledge deficit
   d. Self-esteem disturbance

7. A preschool child who has been burned exhibits a decreased interest in eating. Which of the following measures should the nurse take to increase the child's intake?
   a. Ask the mother to feed the child
   b. Eliminate snacks
   c. Offer smaller and more frequent feedings
   d. Withhold dessert until the meal is eaten

8. A nurse is doing a follow-up assessment of a child who had taken methyl-phenidate (Ritalin) for 1 month. What information should the nurse collect to determine whether the treatment has been effective?
   a. Ask the parents if the child's ability to concentrate and perform tasks has improved
   b. Evaluate head and chest circumference
   c. Ask parents if child's appetite has improved
   d. Assess whether blood pressure has returned to normal

9. An intravenous infusion is started on a child with severe burns. The nurse should assess for signs of fluid overload, which include
   a. Depressed anterior fontanel
   b. Increased abdominal circumference
   c. Moist rales in lung fields
   d. Tea-colored urine

10. An indwelling urinary catheter is inserted into a child with major burns that involve 25% of his body surface area. The nurse informs the parents the primary purpose of this treatment in the emergent phase of burn care is to
    a. Decrease renal workload
    b. Decrease bladder spasm
    c. Prevent urinary retention and infection
    d. Obtain specimens and measure hourly output

ANSWERS, RATIONALES, AND TEST-TAKING TIPS

Rationales	Test-Taking Tips

1. Correct answer: c

A characteristic of some abusive families is inadequate knowledge of normal developmental expectations. A child does not demonstrate physiological and psychological readiness for toilet training until between 18 to 24 months of age. Guilt and anger are expected reactions of parents who blame themselves for their child's illness. The comment in option *b* illustrates a parental method of dealing with the frustrations related to a lack of information about the procedures and treatments for their child. Abusive parents may have fewer support systems and supportive relationships than nonabusive parents.

Reread each of the responses and note that options *a, b,* and *d* are based in reality. Option *c* is different; the statement is a "wish" or "want." Ask if this is a realistic wish; it is not and therefore indicates a need for knowledge of normal child development.

2. Correct answer: c

Children with attention deficit–hyperactivity disorder, AD–HD, benefit from a stable and predictable environment with regular routines and minimal stimuli. Providing rewards for desired behavior should be an immediate action. Although controversial, some children with AD–HD

Approach your choice with an educated guess. Eliminate option *a* because of the key words "use delayed reward." Eliminate option *b*—"processed foods" are commonly inappropriate foods to use. Eliminate option *d*— antidepressant medication is not recommended for AD–HD. Select option *c*.

demonstrate improved behavior when certain processed food additives and artificial colorings are eliminated from their daily diets. Most frequently prescribed medications are sympathomimetic amines, methylphenidate (Ritalin). Antidepressants if used are used sparingly because of cardiac side effects such as tachycardia.

3. Correct answer: c

The diet for a severely burned client must provide sufficient protein and calories to prevent negative nitrogen balance and weight loss. Extra calories should be derived from carbohydrates, because fat sources, although higher in total calories, will not spare protein.

Key words in the stem are "severely burned"—think of a need for high calories. Eliminate options *b* and *d,* which both have fresh vegetables that have minimal calories. Select option *c* over *a,* since option *a* has skim milk, which has less calories.

4. Correct answer: a

As a CNS stimulant, Ritalin's side effects in children and adults include restlessness, insomnia, and tremors. No hematological side effects are associated with Ritalin. A rash, not bleeding or bruising, is the integumentary side effect of Ritalin. Vomiting and diarrhea may occur, but are not the most common side effects.

Recall that Ritalian is a sympathomemitic, which stimulates the central nervous system. The only neurologic findings are in response *a.*

5. Correct answer: c

Besides observable physical evidence of abuse, the type of history revealed by family members or caregivers and their interaction with the child are significant factors in legal proceedings. Therefore, documentation of these observations is essential. The other actions, verbal and mental, are appropriate for the plan of care. However, the priority is written actions; documentation can best be used in court proceedings.

Note the key words "legal proceedings" and associate them with the need for written communication. Cluster the other responses under the category of unwritten communication. Select response c.

6. Correct answer: b

The immediate postburn period, called the emergent phase, is marked by dramatic alteration in circulation. This initial 48 hours postburn is characterized by a decreased cardiac output from a diminished preload, large fluid and plasma protein losses, and edema. The other options are psychosocial needs appropriate for the plan of care for a preschooler with burns. However, physiological needs are the priority in the acute phase of illness or trauma.

Cluster responses a, c, and d under the category of psychological issues. Using Maslow's hierarchy of needs, remember that physiological needs take priority and select response b.

7. Correct answer: c

Serving frequent, smaller meals at least six to seven times daily facilitates the habit of

Small frequent meals are usually a good choice for diet questions.

eating by mouth. The preschool child will typically eat small amounts frequently and prefer finger foods. Many children, especially of preschool age, eat better when they feed themselves. Nourishing snacks should be encouraged to boost caloric intake. Burn clients usually need 5000 to 7000 kcal per day. Meals, including desserts, should provide sufficient protein to prevent negative nitrogen balance.

8. Correct answer: a

Improvement in the ability to concentrate is an appropriate and measurable positive outcome that illustrates the effectiveness of the medication. The other options are not relevant to attention deficit–hyperactivity disorder.

Cluster responses *b, c,* and *d* under the umbrella of physiological growth and function. Response *a* has the focus of mental function improvement, which is different than the other three responses; select response *a.*

9. Correct answer: c

Lung congestion is related to left-sided heart failure secondary to fluid overload. The finding in option *a* is consistent with dehydration and fluid deprivation. The finding in option *b* is consistent with ascites, as in nephrotic syndrome, in which the fluid movement into the interstitial space is secondary to the diminished plasma protein from loss of protein in

Remember *L*ung congestion is related to *L*eft heart failure. The three classic findings for right-sided heart failure are (think of them from the top of the body to the bottom) neck vein distention, hepatomegaly, and edema of the sacral area (if on bed rest) or edema of the feet and ankles. Entire leg edema is typically related to venous or lymphatic dysfunction.

the urine. The finding in option *d* is consistent with acute glomerular nephritis in which the bilirubin is increased in the urine, giving it a brownish color.

10. **Correct answer: d**

Urine volume, measured at least q 1 hour is a priority observation in the emergent phase, the initial 48 hours of burn care, when the primary emphasis is shock prevention. A urine output of 30 cc/hr or ½ cc/kg/ hr is reflective of adequate hydration and cardiac output. The other options are not primary purposes of urinary catheterization for the burn client. In fact, urinary sepsis from indwelling catheters is the most common cause of nosocomial infections.

Associate the priority need to evaluate fluid volume replacement through cardiac output and renal function in the immediate care of burn clients.

Comprehensive Examination

COMPREHENSIVE EXAM QUESTIONS

1. Which of the following is inappropriate to include in the teaching plan for the parent of an infant with iron-deficiency anemia?
   a. Cow's milk and tea increase absorption of iron
   b. Hydrochloric acid (HCl) increases the effectiveness of iron absorption
   c. Proper administration of oral iron supplements
   d. Stool color changes indicate compliance

2. Mrs. Jones, mother of 2-year-old Jeffrey, has received information after he was diagnosed with lead poisoning as a result of eating paint chips. Which of these comments by Mrs. Jones indicates that she needs further instructions?
   a. "Jeffrey will need no follow-up after treatment"
   b. "I will have to give up my leaded glass hobby"
   c. "Lead poisoning may be related to his abnormal eating habits"
   d. "We must leave our house when the walls are being sanded and scraped"

3. A child is to receive calcium disodium edetate (Ca Na$_2$ EDTA). The plan of care should include which of the following items related to assessment?
   a. Daily weights
   b. Erythrocyte protoporphyrin (EP) level
   c. Urinalysis
   d. Complete blood count with a differential white count

4. The nurse obtains all the following data about a 3-year-old child visiting the neighborhood health clinic. About which finding would the nurse be most concerned?
   a. Has not achieved nighttime control of bowel and bladder
   b. Anterior fontanel is open
   c. Constantly asks questions
   d. Cannot draw stickmen but able to copy circles

5. A 3-year-old's mother has been given instructions about pinworm infestation. Which of these statements by the mother indicates the need for no further teaching?
   a. "I'll plan to launder clothes and linens in cold water"
   b. "Lenny cannot be reinfected once he has been treated"
   c. "I'll collect a cellophane tape test after his morning bath"
   d. "I'll encourage Lenny to wash his hands after going to the bathroom and before eating"

6. After receipt of instructions about interventions for infectious mononucleosis, which of these findings indicates the adolescent needs no further teaching?
   a. Frequent contact with persons outside the family during acute phase of illness
   b. Ingestion of aspirin for fever
   c. Regulation of activities according to the degree of shortness of breath
   d. Use of saline gargles to relieve sore throat

7. A child is observed to exhibit seizure activity. Because of this finding, which of these actions by the nursing assistant indicate that the supervisory nurse needs to take corrective action?
   a. Placement of pillows around the child
   b. Insertion of a padded tongue blade or oral airway into the mouth
   c. Prevention of injury to the child from hitting hard or sharp objects
   d. Preparation of the suction equipment

8. An infant's diagnosis is myelomeningocele. To protect the sac from infection, which of these actions by a neophyte registered nurse indicates that the charge nurse needs to do follow-up coaching?
   a. Changed the diapers as soon as they were soiled
   b. Applied a sterile, moist dressing to the sac
   c. Positioned the crib in a low Trendelenburg position
   d. Placed the infant in a prone position at all times

9. The nurse's assessment findings of an infant with the diagnosis of myelomeningocele would probably not include
   a. Dyspnea and cardiac abnormalities
   b. Fecal incontinence and hydrocephalus
   c. Genitourinary and orthopedic abnormalities
   d. Meningeal sac everted and located in the lumbosacral region

10. A child diagnosed with meningitis is restless and irritable when first hospitalized. Which of these initial actions by the student nurse would least promote the child's comfort?
    a. Encouraged the parents to stay with the child
    b. Kept the environmental noise to a minimum
    c. Positioned the child in a side-lying position
    d. Delayed all scheduled testing

11. An infant recently admitted to the pediatric unit has been diagnosed with a patent ductus arteriosus (PDA). When doing a physical assessment of this infant, the nurse should expect which of these findings?
    a. Cyanosis, increased anterior-posterior diameter of chest
    b. Extreme difficulty feeding, irritability
    c. Machinelike murmur, shortness of breath
    d. Systolic murmur, no other significant signs

12. A toddler has been diagnosed as having coarctation of the aorta. Considering the child's diagnosis, the nurse would not anticipate documenting which of these findings?
    a. Weak, thready femoral pulses
    b. Higher blood pressure in the upper extremities
    c. A machinelike murmur
    d. Bounding radial pulses

13. To promote the optimal functioning of a 14-year-old child with hemarthrosis, the nurse instructs a team member to avoid which of the following actions?
    a. Elevate and immobilize the joint in the acute phase
    b. Institute passive range of motion to the joint after the acute phase
    c. Apply pressure to the area for 10 to 15 minutes
    d. Apply warm compresses to the joint

14. Which of these instructions given by the neophyte nurse to the parents concerning their child who is recovering from a sickle cell crisis is inaccurate information?
    a. Avoid contact with all children
    b. Isolate child from known sources of infection
    c. Allow as desired fluid intake including requests for fluids during the night
    d. Reinforce the basics of trait transmission

15. A 10-year-old child with a severe asthma attack is brought to the emergency room by his parents. Considering the child's diagnosis, the child would most likely have had which of these findings as a prodromal symptom?
    a. Hacking, nonproductive cough
    b. Itching at base of neck or over upper back
    c. Shortness of breath, prolonged expiratory phase
    d. Mild, inspiratory wheezing

16. Eight-year-old Gina is admitted to the pediatric unit with a respiratory infection. She was diagnosed with cystic fibrosis as an infant. The physician orders all of the following medications for Gina. Which one should the nurse question?
    a. Theodur
    b. Robitussin with codeine
    c. Mucomyst
    d. Phazyme

17. The parents receive instructions regarding chest physiotherapy. Which of the following statements by the parent indicates the need for no further teaching?
    a. "I'll start a nebulizer treatment after chest physiotherapy"
    b. "I'll plan to do chest physiotherapy after breakfast"
    c. "I plan to do percussion and vibration during postural drainage"
    d. "Chest physiotherapy must be done only when needed"

18. Following a tonsillectomy in a child, the nurse suspects hemorrhage at the operative site. Which of these findings should the nursing assistant report to the nurse promptly?
    a. Cold skin, progressive cyanosis, sweating
    b. Pulse of 100, constant complaints of the throat hurting, increased restlessness
    c. Temperature of 100° F, pulse of 100, respiratory rate of 24
    d. Discomfort when swallowing, clammy skin, pale color

19. A 3-year-old child is brought to the emergency room with the following symptoms: fever, restlessness, and drooling. No coughing is observed. Based on these findings, which of the following activities should the nurse instruct the student nurse to do?
    a. Continuously monitor the airway status
    b. Examine the throat with a tongue depressor
    c. Take a throat culture
    d. Prepare antibiotics for immediate infusion

20. An infant has undergone surgical repair of bilateral cleft lip. Which of these goals is least important in the infant's immediate care?
    a. Adequate hydration is provided
    b. The family is supported
    c. Trauma to suture line is prevented
    d. Operative site remains free of infection

21. A staff member includes all of the following measures in caring for an infant who has had cleft lip repair surgery. Which of these actions indicates that the staff member needs no additional coaching?
    a. Infant is placed in elbow restraints
    b. Infant is placed in prone position to facilitate drainage of secretions
    c. Infant's suture line is cleansed gently every 8 hours
    d. Both restraints are removed simultaneously

22. A parent receives preoperative instructions for an infant who is diagnosed with pyloric stenosis. Which of these statements by the parent indicates inadequate knowledge of the instructions?
    a. "Feeding with formula may begin 6 hours after surgery"
    b. "Feeding with glucose water may begin 6 hours after surgery"
    c. "The baby will be fed during the first 24 hours after surgery"
    d. "The baby will be started on clear fluids immediately after surgery"

23. The charge nurse expects that the team member caring for an infant who has had a pyloromyotomy will not position the infant in which of the following ways?
    a. In a fowler's position
    b. In a prone position on a pillow
    c. On the right side after feeding
    d. On the right side while lying in a car seat

24. An infant is admitted to the hospital with a report by the parents of sudden episodes of drawing up the legs as if having acute abdominal pain. Which of the following questions by the admission nurse would elicit the most essential information if the physician suspects intussusception?
    a. "How frequent are the episodes?"
    b. "Has the infant had projectile vomiting?"
    c. "Does the stool look like currant jelly?"
    d. "Do you burp the child frequently while feeding?"

25. A preschooler is brought to the pediatrician's office because of a fever and very irritable behavior. The child is diagnosed with a urinary tract infection. Which of the following statements is inappropriate to document in the teaching plan related to Bactrim?
    a. Avoid exposure to the sun when taking Bactrim
    b. Do not discontinue the medications when the symptoms disappear
    c. Have the child drink at least 4 to 6 ounces of fluid with each administration of Bactrim
    d. The medication will turn the urine orange

26. A 6-year-old child has been diagnosed with acute glomerulonephritis. Considering the diagnosis, which of the following findings documented by the student nurse is probably an error in the notes?
   a. Elevated blood pressure and anorexia
   b. Periorbital edema and grossly bloody urine
   c. Severe anasarca and ascites
   d. Oliguria with cloudy, hematuric characteristics

27. With a medical diagnosis of nephrotic syndrome, which of these nursing diagnoses is least important?
   a. Fluid volume excess
   b. Risk for impaired skin integrity
   c. Risk for injury
   d. Activity intolerance

28. A parent has been given instructions about a Pavlik harness to be worn by an infant with congenital hip dysplasia. Which of these statements by the parent would need to be reported by the nursing assistant to the registered nurse?
   a. "We don't plan to remove the harness unless approved by the physician"
   b. "We'll make follow-up appointments for harness readjustment"
   c. "We must maintain the hips in an out-from-the-body position"
   d. "We can remove the harness for diaper changes"

29. An 18-month-old child is scheduled for application of plaster cast to correct a clubfoot. Which of the following measures would be inappropriate to include in the postoperative plan of care?
   a. Elevate the cast to at or above the level of the heart when the child is in a lying position
   b. Handle the cast without the use of the fingertips
   c. Reposition the child every 2 hours
   d. Spray the cast with acrylic

30. After performing a physical assessment of a 12-year-old client, the nurse should document which of these findings related to scoliosis?
   a. Asymmetry of shoulders, back, and waist
   b. Convex angulation in thoracic area
   c. Concave curvature of lumbar spine
   d. Malformation of vertebrae

31. Which of the following statements by a parent indicates knowledge of why an infant must wear a Pavlik harness?
    a. "It provides comfort and support"
    b. "It shortens the limb on the bad side"
    c. "It maintains the long bone in the upper leg within its socket"
    d. "It provides outward movement of the head of the long bone in the leg"

32. Which of these assessments of a child with a cast for correction of clubfoot is a priority for the care technician to report?
    a. The cast has not dried in 8 to 12 hours
    b. The recent check results are color change of the toes and cool skin proximal to cast
    c. Client moves toes and capillary refill is less than 4.5 seconds
    d. Rough edges are found on the cast

33. A school-age child diagnosed with juvenile diabetes has been taught the importance of site rotation for insulin administration. Which of these statements made by the child indicates a need for no further teaching?
    a. "I won't use a site that contains bulges"
    b. "Once I find a comfortable site, I'll use it frequently"
    c. "I must record the site of my insulin injections on a weekly basis"
    d. "I may only use the abdomen and arms for self-injections and never my thighs"

34. The nurse is planning to teach the mother of an infant diagnosed with hypothyroidism about proper administration of levothyroxine (Synthroid). Which of the following guidelines documented on the teaching plan of how to mix the crushed medication is incorrect?
    a. Mix with 4 ounces of formula in a bottle
    b. Mix with 5 cc of cherry syrup
    c. Mix in a very small amount of baby food
    d. Mix in 1 teaspoonful of baby cereal mixed with applesauce

35. A 7-year-old child is diagnosed with attention deficit–hyperactivity disorder (AD–HD). To promote the child's optimal functioning, which of these approaches should be avoided?
    a. Encourage the use of an immediate reward system
    b. Encourage a diet that emphasizes processed foods
    c. Place the child in a structured, small classroom environment
    d. Obtain a prescription for sympathomimetic medications

36. The team member admits an 18-month-old child with multiple extremity fractures. This is the child's third admission in 3 months for fractures. Which comment by the mother should be reported by the team member to the nurse in charge?
    a. "I blame myself for this injury"
    b. "I want to know what is going to be done for my child"
    c. "I wish my child would be potty trained"
    d. "My sister helps care for my child"

37. A rapid intravenous infusion is started on a newly admitted infant with severe burns. The student nurse would most likely document which of the following findings on the admission assessment form?
    a. Depressed anterior fontanel
    b. Increased abdominal circumference
    c. Moist rales in lung fields
    d. Tea-colored urine

38. A mother has been given instructions regarding the administration of pediatric digoxin (Lanoxin). The physician has ordered the medication to be administered BID. Which of these statements by the parent indicates a need for more instructions?
    a. "I'll give the medication with breakfast and lunch"
    b. "I'll mix the medication with a teaspoon of applesauce"
    c. "I won't give another dose if the baby vomits"
    d. "I'll give the medication before meals, 12 hours apart"

39. Which of the following statements given by a school-age child's parent indicates that the child is at risk for developing chicken pox?
    a. "My child complains of a sore throat"
    b. "Bluish-white 'spots' are in the child's mouth"
    c. "My child has a runny nose, 99° F temperature, and feels tired"
    d. "My child played with friends, one of whom had the chicken pox and didn't know it at the time"

ANSWERS, RATIONALES, AND TEST-TAKING TIPS

Rationales	Test-Taking Tips

1. Correct answer: a

Tannins in tea form an insoluble iron complex. HCl acid enhances effectiveness of iron, because it helps reduce iron to its most soluble state. Oral iron supplements are administered daily in two divided doses. Stool color change to dark green or black would indicate compliance with administration of prescribed medication.

Caution is necessary in this type of question to zero in on the key word "inappropriate." If the question is read quickly, the incorrect selection may be made. A better process is to read the question, read the responses, *then* reread the question followed with the reading of your selected answer to ensure that you have made the correct choice.

2. Correct answer: a

Follow-up monitoring after treatment is necessary to assess efficacy of the treatment. Hobbies such as making leaded glass windows introduce lead into the home. Therefore, Mrs. Jones would be commended for the pursuit of another hobby besides leaded glass until her son is older. Abnormal eating of nonfood substances (pica) may contributes to lead ingestion. The deleading process—sanding and scraping of painted surfaces—contributes to significant amounts of ingested and inhaled lead for the home's inhabitants.

Quick reading may result in an incorrect answer. If the focus of "need for further teaching" is overlooked, and instead you read or think of the question as "no further teaching needed," an answer will be selected that indicates adequate knowledge. The correct answer to this question will involve relaying inadequate knowledge.

3. Correct answer: b

EP level is part of the diagnostic workup before the treatment for lead poisoning. CBC with a differential white count is useful in determining evidence of anemia and/or infection. It does not typically reflect any evaluation of glomeruli filtration function. Weight is the best indicator of overall fluid balance. Since Ca Na$_2$ EDTA and lead are both toxic to the kidneys, records of I&O are frequently kept. A urinalysis is performed to evaluate general renal functioning. A serum creatinine test best evaluates renal function, but it is not given as a choice.

If the answer is unknown, cluster responses *a*, *c*, and *d* under the focus of more general assessments and select response *b*, which is a specific test.

4. Correct answer: b

The anterior fontanel should have closed at age 18 months. Nighttime bowel and bladder control may be achieved by 3 years of age; some children may take longer than 3 years. Preschoolers typically ask many questions, particularly "why." The behavior in option *d* is consistent with a 3-year-old's ability.

If you have no idea of the correct response, cluster the responses into those of nonphysical examination, options *a*, *c*, and *d*; select the physical examination, option *b*.

5. Correct answer: d

Handwashing after toileting and before eating prevents reinfection; laundering clothes and linens in hot

The first step is to correctly read and comprehend what the question is asking—"need for no further teaching." In reading the

water prevents reinfection. Reinfection is possible due to easy transmission and ability to survive for up to one week in the environment. The cellophane tape test for pinworm specimens is collected in the morning before the child awakens and before the child bathes or has a bowel movement.

responses, a statement of adequate knowledge should be selected. Do not forget, once you have selected an option, to reread the question and your selection. Words in each response that clue to an incorrect answer are in *a*: "cold water," in *b*: "cannot be reinfected," and in *c*: "after . . . bath."

6. Correct answer: d

A sore throat is relieved by saline gargles, hot drinks, or warm water. Outside contact increases the risk of secondary infections; therefore, it should be limited. A mild analgesic is usually sufficient to relieve headache, fever, and malaise. However, this is a teen and ASA should not be given because of the risk of Reye's syndrome. Affected individuals should be instructed to regulate their activity level to tolerance. Respiratory problems are typically not included in the sequela of mononucleosis. Bed rest is encouraged for complaints of fatigue.

The phrase "needs no further teaching" guides to the selection of answer *d*. Option *a* can be eliminated, since common sense dictates that a sick person is not to have frequent contact with others. Eliminate response *c*, since mononucleosis is characterized more commonly by fatigue and headaches, not shortness of breath.

7. Correct answer: b

Force should not be exerted in an attempt to place solid objects between teeth to maintain an airway, especially during a seizure. Airways are

The actions that require no corrective follow-up by the nurse, options *a*, *c*, and *d*, can be clustered as actions that protect and prevent injury to the client.

only appropriate if inserted
before the beginning of a
seizure, but the child must
be protected from injury
during the seizure, but the
convulsing client should not
be restrained during a
seizure. Suction may be
needed after the seizure
activity has stopped.

8. Correct answer: d

Option *d* is incorrect because of
the phrase "all the time";
rather than a true prone
position, the position
suggested is more of a side-
lying or semiprone position.
Myelomeningocele sac must
remain free of urine or stool
contamination; therefore,
frequent diaper changes are
essential. It is more often
located in the low thoracic,
lumbar, or sacral region.
Dressings applied to the sac
are moistened, usually with
sterile normal saline, to
prevent drying of the sac.
Ideally, the infant is placed in
low Trendelenburg position to
reduce spinal fluid pressure in
the sac, with hips flexed to
avoid pressure on the defect.
Range of motion to the lower
extremities is needed daily to
prevent flexion contractures.

Most often, options such as *d* that
contain absolutes are incorrect.
Note that the question is asking
for an incorrect action, since there
is a need for follow-up coaching.

9. Correct answer: a

Findings of cardiac and
pulmonary difficulties are not
consistent with neural tube
defect. Fecal incontinence

The question is asking what is not
to be expected in a neurological
abnormality—"meningo" gives a
clue that it is a nerve. Of the given

and hydrocephalus are the most frequent characteristics evident in myelomeningocele. Myelomeningocele is one of the most common causes of neurogenic bladder. Orthopedic anomalies of the hip, knee, and foot are all possibilities and depend on the location of the spinal lesion. The largest number of defects are located in the lumbar or lumbosacral region.

options, responses *b*, *c*, and *d* have neurological tones and response *a* does not; select it.

10. Correct answer: d

Acute meningitis is a medical emergency. Early recognition of causative organisms through tests is necessary to begin immediate antibiotic therapy for the prevention of death or disability. Parents should be encouraged to stay with the child and become involved in the care to decrease separation anxiety and minimize psychological trauma. The room should be kept as quiet as possible and environmental stimuli kept at a minimum, since most children are sensitive to noise, bright lights, and other environmental stimuli. All of these stimuli have potential to increase intracranial pressure. The child should be positioned in a side-lying position because of nuchal rigidity, which is characterized by neck hyperextension. Children will usually assume this position naturally.

If you have no idea of the correct response, cluster responses *a*, *b*, and *d* under the focus of direct actions for comfort. Select response *d*, which doesn't promote comfort; if the tests are delayed, the diagnosis and treatment will be delayed, ultimately interfering with the child's comfort.

11. Correct answer: c

The findings of a machinelike murmur and shortness of breath are consistent with patent ductus arteriosus—the turbulent flow of blood from the aorta through the PDA to the pulmonary artery results in a characteristic machinery like murmur. The findings in option *a* are consistent with cystic fibrosis. In option *b* the findings are consistent with congestive heart failure and/or a gastrointestinal condition. One of the characteristic signs of ventricular septal defect is a loud, harsh, pansystolic murmur heard best at the lower left sternal border.

Look for key words in each option to eliminate incorrect choices: in option *a* "cyanosis and chest diameter" are too general to answer a question about a specific abnormality; in option *b* the word "extreme" clues that feeding has no relationship to a vascular problem; and in option *c*, "no other significant signs" is again too general to be the answer to a specific question.

12. Correct answer: c

A characteristic of patent ductus arteriosus is the finding in option c. Femoral pulses, which are distal to the defect, are weak or absent in coarctation of the aorta. Coarctation of the aorta (COA) is first assessed at a routine physical examination with upper extremity hypertension. In those body areas that receive blood from vessels proximal to the defect, the BP is high and the pulses are bounding.

Key words in the stem are "the aorta" and "would not anticipate." If the aorta has a problem, a murmur is unlikely, since murmurs are caused by turbulent blood flow, usually from dysfunctional valves in the heart.

13. Correct answer: d

Cold packs or compresses promote vasoconstriction and should be used instead of warm compresses, which dilate the vessels. The warm compresses would promote more bleeding. During bleeding episodes, the joint is elevated and immobilized to prevent crippling effects of joint degeneration. This action is specific to hemarthrosis. Passive range of motion exercises are instituted after the acute phase. Pressure to the area must be applied for at least 10 to 15 minutes to allow for clot formation.

Use common sense to select response *d*, which would increase bleeding.

14. Correct answer: a

Parents must understand the need to balance the developmental needs of the child and the need for living a normal life. Since infection is a major predisposing factor in the development of a physiologic crisis and the body's immune system is compromised, the parents should understand the need to isolate the child from sources of infection. Hydration is necessary for hemodilution, which prevents sickling; therefore, fluids are not restricted, even at night. Option *d* is an appropriate intervention after the initial diagnosis and during follow-up.

The absolute, "all," in response *a* clues the reader that this is probably the incorrect response. Don't stop after reading option *a*, or an incorrect selection may be made. If you have a pattern of selecting options *a* or *b* and not reading all the options, try reading backwards—from *d* up to *a*—to more clearly comprehend all the words, quickly detect key words, and resist the temptation to not read some options.

15. Correct answer: b

Itching at the base of the neck or over the upper back is observed as the prodromal symptom, the first indicator of the onset of a disease. Asthma attacks begin with a hacking, nonproductive cough. A child with a severe asthma attack is short of breath and tries to breathe more deeply. The expiratory phase becomes prolonged and is accompanied by auditory wheezing. Wheezing usually occurs on expiration in asthma attacks.

If you have no idea of the correct response, cluster responses *a, c,* and *d* under respiratory findings and select response *b,* a nonrespiratory finding.

16. Correct answer: b

Codeine is an antitussive, a cough suppressant. Increased viscosity of respiratory secretions contributes to the risk of infection. Coughing moves secretions to facilitate expectoration and, therefore, decreases the risk of infection. A medication that inhibits coughing should be questioned. Bronchodilators are appropriately ordered via nebulizer to open the bronchi for easier expectoration. Mucolytic agents are used to decrease the viscosity of mucous secretions or relieve meconium ileus. Pancreatic enzymes are administered with meals and snacks to ensure that these digestive enzymes are mixed with food in the duodenum.

In cystic fibrosis the exocrine secretions are thick; these secretions include mucus of the respiratory tract and the pancreatic secretions.

17. Correct answer: c

Chest physiotherapy includes the use of postural drainage in combination with the adjunct techniques of percussion and vibration, which are believed to enhance mucus movement and removal from the airway. Bronchodilator medication in an aerosol helps open bronchi for easier expectoration and is done before chest physiotherapy. Chest physiotherapy is generally performed before meals to minimize the chance of vomiting. Chest physiotherapy is usually performed twice daily and more frequently if the child has a respiratory infection.

In order to get this question correct, you must read slowly and accurately. The question requires adequate knowledge as depicted in the phrase "need for no further teaching."

18. Correct answer: b

The subtle early sign is the child's continuous complaints of the throat hurting from continuous swallowing of trickling blood down the back of the throat. Airway obstruction is indicated by progressive cyanosis. Cold skin and the appearance of sweating may be environmental, since humidifiers are used to decrease the drying of the mucous membranes. The findings in option *c* are not consistent with hemorrhage. Option *d* is a false statement; discomfort is expected following this surgery.

The clue in the stem is "hemorrhage." The clues in the option *b* are "constant" complaints, which indirectly indicate that the client is frequently swallowing with bleeding. The other clue is the classic finding in the initial stage of shock—increased "restlessness." Note in response *d* that discomfort when swallowing is an expected finding.

19. Correct answer: a

Three clinical observations that have been known to predict epiglottitis are the absence of a spontaneous cough, the presence of drooling, and agitation. Continuous monitoring of the respiratory status is a priority. When epiglottitis is suspected, nurses should not attempt to visualize the epiglottis or take a throat culture. Assessment of the respiratory status is the priority.

Eliminate responses *b*, *c*, and *d* since these are interventions; with application of the nursing process it is best to do further assessment before interventions. Response *d* is also incorrect, since no data exist in the stem to indicate that a culture was done, which is needed before initial antibiotic administration.

20. Correct answer: d

Option *d* is an appropriate goal in the postsugical period for the child with cleft lip repair; however, it is least important in the immediate care, within a few hours after the return from surgery. Protection from trauma is a more immediate concern. Hydration is achieved with IVs until the child takes fluids by mouth. Hydration is important to maintain the cardiac output. Physiological needs of the infant take priority in the immediate postoperative period along with care of the parents' psychological needs. If these parental needs are ignored, the parents' anxiety may be transferred to the infant. A major priority in the postsurgical period is protection of the operative site to ensure optimum healing and cosmetic repair.

Cluster responses *a*, *b*, and *c* under the goals that directly affect the client and option *d*, a nonclient goal, is least important.

21. Correct answer: a

Use of elbow restraints is recommended to prevent the infant from rubbing the incision. An infant who has had cleft lip repair must be prevented from lying on the abdomen and rubbing the face on the sheets. To prevent infection and enhance healing, the suture line is cleansed of formula as needed after feedings. Removal of restraints one at a time allows for exercise of the arms and allows for stimulation and body contact. However, the restraints would not be removed together, since it would be too hard to control both arms at the same time.

Look for the correct action: "needs no further coaching." Prone position facilitates drainage; however, it also promotes irritation of the suture line. Cleansing of the suture line of an area that has frequent secretions is typically done as needed, PRN.

22. Correct answer: a

Clear fluids are instituted before formula to establish tolerance. Postsurgical feedings are usually instituted relatively soon. They usually begin with clear liquids that contain glucose and electrolytes. Feedings with formula are instituted within 24 hours, unless contraindicated.

Look for an incorrect answer, since the question is asking for "inadequate knowledge." Read carefully and use the following process on these types of questions: read the question and options, select your option, and reread the question and then your choice of option to confirm it to be the correct one.

23. Correct answer: b

Option *b* is the correct positioning for an infant with *gastroesophageal reflux*. The infant, after a

The caution here is to read the question carefully—"to not position" the infant in which manner.

pyloromyotomy, is positioned in high fowler's, also called fowler's, and slightly on the right side after feeding to facilitate gastric emptying. High fowler's is preferred to decrease the risk of vomiting and aspiration.

24. Correct answer: c

As intussusception progresses, the affected infant demonstrates increased vomiting, apathy, and passage of stools mixed with blood and mucus, which give the stool a currant-jelly consistency. The frequency of the episodes adds no essential information to the assessment data. Although vomiting, not usually projectile, is associated with this and a number of other gastrointestinal conditions, the passage of currant-jelly–type stool is most characteristic of intussusception. This disease process is not linked to feeding technique; it is a structural abnormality of the intestine in which one segment of the intestine telescopes or prolapses into the lumen of another segment. A barium enema is usually used to confirm the diagnosis.

The key words in the stem are "sudden episodes" and "intussusception" or telescoping of the intestine, which would result in an irritation and possibly bleeding. Eliminate responses *a* and *d*, since they are too general for the specific question. Projectile vomiting is classic in pyloric valve stenosis and increased intracranial pressure.

25. Correct answer: d

Option *d* is a side effect of Pyridium (phenazopyridine hydrochloride), a local urinary analgesic that soothes the mucosa of the urinary tract to eliminate the burning with urination found in urinary tract infections. Sulfonamides such as Bactrim produce photosensitivity; the child should avoid exposure to ultraviolet light and direct sunlight. Urinary medications, like other antibiotics, should be administered for the entire course of therapy, not until symptoms disappear. Any medication given for urinary tract infections should be administered with adequate fluids to facilitate the elimination of crystals that result from the action of the medication. If sufficient fluids are not given, these crystals can form stones in the kidneys.

If you have no idea of the correct response, select option *d* since common sense dictates that compared to the other given answers it is the least important; it is not a finding with this medication.

26. Correct answer: c

The findings in option *c* are consistent with nephrotic syndrome. Anasarca is generalized edema and ascites is edema of the abdominal area. In acute glomerulonephritis (AGN), the BP is mildly to moderately increased and anorexia is a major gastrointestinal finding. In

Note the important characteristic in the stem—"an acute" problem. In the responses, "severe" anasarca and ascites are typically found in "chronic" pathologic situations. This documentation of anasarca and ascites indicates an error.

AGN, decreased plasma filtration results in an excessive accumulation of water and sodium retention. Initial signs include puffiness of the face, especially around the eyes (called periorbital edema), and the passage of dark-colored urine, which may be described as wine (red) colored. This is different from the tea-colored or yellow-brownish colored urine that has bilirubin in it from liver and gallbladder problems such as obstructed bile ducts as a result of gallstones. Cloudy urine is from proteinuria. Oliguria and hematuria are classic findings in AGN.

27. Correct answer: c

Risk for injury is more appropriate in the chronic stage of kidney failure when neurological physiology is most affected. Regular evaluations of intake, output, and body weight are essential to monitor fluid balance and disease progression. Skin care is a major consideration in children with nephrotic syndrome in which the edema is typically generalized and severe. Fatigue is commonly associated with nephrotic syndrome.

Note that all of the responses are correct. Select the one that is on the bottom of the list, after you have prioritized the items.

28. Correct answer: d

Diapering may be accomplished without harness removal. The physician may or may not allow the harness's removal for bathing. The infant should be examined by the practitioner before any adjustment is attempted to make certain the hips are in correct placement before the harness is resecured. A Pavlik harness is used to maintain the hip in abducted position.

The reading process is important with this type of question. Read the stem, the options, select an option, reread the question, reread your selection, and confirm it is the focus of the question.

29. Correct answer: d

Option *d* is not an appropriate action. Turning the child every 2 hours will help dry the cast evenly. Drying can take up to 72 hours if traditional plaster materials are used. Casted extremities should be elevated on a pillow to increase venous return, minimize edema, and provide comfort. The damp cast should be handled by the palms of the hands to prevent indenting the cast. Indentations can create pressure areas under the cast.

Reading is important to correct answer selection. Don't miss *in*appropriate—look for an incorrect action.

30. Correct answer: a

Rib, hump, and flank asymmetry cause imbalances of the shoulders, back, and waist. Option *b* is a definition for kyphosis. Option *c* is a

Associate scoliosis with shoulder symmetry problems.

definition for lordosis. Scoliosis involves a spinal curvature and is not associated with a vertebrae problem.

31. Correct answer: c

The Pavlik harness works with gravity to move the hip into a more abducted position, with the proximal femur centered in the acetabulum. Positioning is the primary purpose of the harness, not comfort and support. Options *b* and *d* are not purposes of this harness. Note that leg shortening on the affected side is a finding consistent with congenital dislocated hip.

Look for correct knowledge. Use common sense to eliminate options *b* (bones are not to be shortened) and *d* (when the head of the femur moves outward it becomes dislocated). Reread the question— it is a specific question about a specific treatment. Of the remaining responses, *c* is more specific than the general option *a*, so select option *c* as the correct response.

32. Correct answer: b

Any proximal or distal discoloration of a casted extremity or change in neurovascular status needs to be reported promptly to the nurse assigned to the client. Options *a*, *c*, and *d* are normal findings that are important to report; however, abnormal findings should be reported first. Casts made of traditional materials, plaster of paris, may take up to 72 hours before completely dried. Raw edges of the cast can be protected by petaling the edges with tape.

Cluster options *a*, *c*, and *d* under concerns about the cast; eliminate these as choices. In comparison, option *b* is a concern about a change in the client's status; it is the priority and therefore the correct answer.

33. **Correct answer: a**

The child should avoid sites with fat pads, bulges, that develop in overused areas. Fat pads may develop if one site is continuously injected. Recording site of insulin injection on a daily basis is emphasized to prevent overutilization of one site and to have a more accurate record as compared to recording sites once a week. Appropriate sites for self-injection of insulin are the abdomen and arms; however, the thighs can also be used.

Read carefully; look for a correct statement or knowledge of the right action. There are words in the options that guide you to eliminate them as the best answer: in option *b* "frequently"; in option *c* "record . . . weekly"; and in option *d* "only use . . . never." Absolutes such as *only* or *never* are clues to an incorrect answer in most cases.

34. **Correct answer: a**

Medication is not mixed in formula in a bottle, since control for the amount given would be difficult. Flavored syrup is an acceptable medium in which to mix crushed medication. Crushed medications should be mixed with 1 teaspoon of a sweet-tasting substance such as applesauce.

Cluster responses *b*, *c*, and *d* under the size of small amounts and eliminate, since the question is asking for an incorrect action.

35. **Correct answer: b**

This approach is controversial and should not be used routinely. Some children with AD–HD demonstrate improved behavior when certain processed food

If you have narrowed the responses to *b* and *d*, reread the question and these two responses. Option *b* is less documented as effective for children with AD–HD overall and is the best answer.

additives and artificial colorings are eliminated. Providing rewards for desired behavior should be an immediate action. Children with AD–HD benefit from a stable and predictable environment with regular routines and in which stimuli are reduced to a minimum. The most frequently prescribed medications are sympathomimetic amines-methylphenidate (Ritalin). Antidepressants are used sparingly because of cardiac side effects.

36. Correct answer: c

A characteristic of some abusive families is inadequate knowledge of normal developmental expectations. A child does not demonstrate physiological and psychological readiness for toilet training until 18 to 24 months of age. Some children are even later than these given guidelines. Guilt and anger are expected reactions of most parents as they blame themselves for their child's illness. The comment in option *b* is a method of dealing with frustrations related to the lack of information about procedures and treatment. Abusive families often have fewer supportive relationships with extended families and friends than nonabusive parents.

If you have no idea of the correct answer, cluster options *a, b,* and *c* under the focus of reality. In option *c,* "I wish" is a clue for a nonreality-based statement. Select it as the best choice.

37. Correct answer: a

Option *a* is consistent with vascular dehydration, which occurs within the first 24 to 48 hours in severe burns. Option *b* is consistent with ascites, as in nephrotic syndrome and has nothing to do with burns. Option *c* is a consistent finding in fluid overload, which is the greatest risk in after the initial 48 hours of therapy. The finding in option *d* is consistent with acute glomerulonephritis.

Note that the term "severe burns" may be a distractor. The question is inquiring about what might be a finding on the initial assessment of the infant.

38. Correct answer: a

Digoxin is given 1 hour before or 2 hours after feedings; this would be on an empty stomach. Digoxin administration guidelines include giving the medication at regular intervals (usually 12 hours apart). Medication is mixed with a small amount of a sweet substance to control and ensure the medication is taken. If the child vomits, digoxin guidelines indicate a second dose should not be given.

Read the question and options slowly and carefully. Look for incorrect information, since the question is asking for "a need for more instruction."

39. Correct answer: d

Transmission of varicella is by direct contact with skin lesions or, more commonly, by droplets spread from the respiratory tract of infected persons, usually in the prodromal period or the

The key words in the stem are "at risk" for the disease. If you had no idea of the correct response, match the disease "chicken pox" in the stem with the response that has the words in it, option *d*.

early stages of the rash. The
vesicular fluid and the scabs
are infectious until entirely
dry. Incubation period lasts
2 to 3 weeks, followed by a
slight fever, mild headache,
malaise, and anorexia,
occurring about 24 to 36
hours before the rash
begins. The lesions, which
are typically in all stages
simultaneously, erupt first on
the back and chest and then
spread to the face, neck, and
limbs. They typically are not
on the soles of the feet or
the palms of the hands.
Option *a* is consistent with
bacterial infection of the
throat or rubella. Spots with
bluish-white center (Koplik)
are associated with rubeola.
The findings in option *c* of
upper respiratory infection
are not consistent with the
usual mode of disease
progression.

BIBLIOGRAPHY

Advisory Committee on Immunization Practices: General recommendations on immunizations, *MMWR* 43(RR-1), 1994.

American Academy of Pediatrics, Committee on Genetics: Folic acid for the prevention of neural tube defects. *Pediatrics* 92(3):493-494, 1993.

American Academy of Pediatrics: *Report of the committee on infectious diseases,* ed 22, Elk Grove, Ill., 1991.

Betz CL and Poster EC: *Mosby's pediatric nursing reference,* ed 2, St Louis, 1992, Mosby.

Chess S and Thomas A: Temperamental differences: a critical concept in child health care, *Pediatric Nursing* 11:167-171, 1985.

Erikson E: *Childhood and society,* New York, 1963, W.W. Norton.

Erikson E: *Identity: youth and crisis,* New York, 1968, W.W. Norton.

Hazinski M: Cardiovascular disorders. In Hazinski M, editor: *Nursing care of the critically ill child,* ed 2, St Louis, 1992, Mosby.

Jackson DB and Saunders RB: *Child health nursing,* Philadelphia, 1993, J.B. Lippincott.

Jaffe M: *Pediatric nursing care plans,* El Paso, 1993, Skidmore-Roth.

Piaget J: *The theory of stages of cognitive development,* New York, 1969, McGraw-Hill.

Rollant, P. Acing multiple choice tests, *AJN Career Guide,* Jan: 18-21, 36, 1994.

Seidel HM et al: *Mosby's guide to physical examination,* St Louis, 1991, Mosby.

Tanner J: Issues and advances in adolescent growth and development, *Journal of Adolescent Health Care* 8:470-478, 1987.

Whaley L and Wong D: *Nursing care of infants and children,* ed 4, St Louis, 1991, Mosby.

Wong, D: *Whaley and Wong's nursing care of infants and children,* ed 5, St Louis, 1995, Mosby.

Wong D: *Essentials of pediatric nursing,* ed 4, St Louis, 1993, Mosby.

INDEX

Instructions for Disk Start-Up

DOS Version
System Requirements

A computer with at least 324K of RAM (Random Access Memory) available is needed for this program. This computer must be IBM PC or 100% compatible.

For these examples we assume that your A drive is your floppy drive, and your C drive is your hard drive. Please substitute the letter of your floppy drive for A if your floppy drive letter is different. Substitute the letter of your hard drive for C if your hard drive letter is different.

Start-up (floppy drive):

1. Turn your computer on
2. At the prompt, insert the disk into your A drive
3. Type A: and press <Enter>
4. Type MOSBY and press <Enter>
5. Follow the instructions on the screen

Start-up (hard disk):

1. Turn your computer on
2. At the prompt, insert the disk into your A drive
3. Type C: and press <Enter>
4. Type MD\MOSBY and press <Enter>
5. Type CD\MOSBY and press <Enter>
6. Type COPY A:*.* and press <Enter>

The software is now installed on your hard drive. Once the software is installed, start the software by following these directions:

1. Type CD\MOSBY and press <Enter>
2. Type MOSBY and press <Enter>
3. Follow the directions on the screen

MAC Version

System Requirements

Mac 68XXX or Power Mac with a total of at least 1 MB of RAM is needed for this program.

Start-up:

1. Create a new folder on your hard disk called MOSBY.
2. Insert the disk into your floppy drive and open it.
3. Drag all items from the disk to the new folder.

The software is now installed on your hard drive. Once the software is installed, start the software by following these directions:

1. Open the MOSBY folder.
2. Select the MOSBY program.
3. Follow the directions on the screen.

WRITE DOWN THE PASSWORD THAT YOU HAVE SELECTED.
YOUR DISK WILL BE BRANDED WITH THIS INITIAL ENTRY.